Practical Case Studies in Hypertension Management

Series Editor
Giuliano Tocci
Rome, Italy

The aim of the book series "Practical Case Studies in Hypertension Management" is to provide physicians who treat hypertensive patients having different cardiovascular risk profiles with an easy-to-access tool that will enhance their clinical practice, improve average blood pressure control, and reduce the incidence of major hypertension-related complications. To achieve these ambitious goals, each volume presents and discusses a set of paradigmatic clinical cases relating to different scenarios in hypertension. These cases will serve as a basis for analyzing best practice and highlight problems in implementing the recommendations contained in international guidelines regarding diagnosis and treatment. While the available guidelines have contributed significantly in improving the diagnostic process, cardiovascular risk stratification, and therapeutic management in patients with essential hypertension, they are of limited help to physicians in daily clinical practice when approaching individual patients with hypertension, and this is particularly true when choosing among different drug classes and molecules. By discussing exemplary clinical cases that may better represent clinical practice in a "real world" setting, this series will assist physicians in selecting the best diagnostic and therapeutic options.

More information about this series at
http://www.springer.com/series/13624

Arrigo F.G. Cicero

Hypertension and Metabolic Cardiovascular Risk Factors

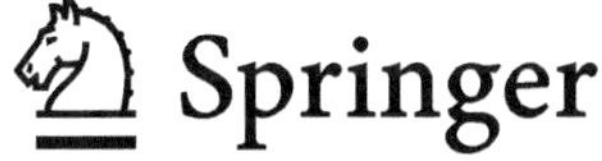

Arrigo F.G. Cicero
S Orsola-Malpighi Hospital
Cardiovascular Disease Prevention Research Unit
Via Albertoni 15
40138 Bologna
Bologna
Italy

ISSN 2364-6632 ISSN 2364-6640 (electronic)
Practical Case Studies in Hypertension Management
ISBN 978-3-319-39503-6 ISBN 978-3-319-39504-3 (eBook)
DOI 10.1007/978-3-319-39504-3

Library of Congress Control Number: 2016944619

Printed on acid-free paper

This Springer imprint is published by Springer Nature
The registered company is Springer International Publishing AG Switzerland

Foreword

Essential hypertension is frequently associated with various metabolic abnormalities, such as fasting glucose impairment, hyperglycemia, diabetes, visceral obesity, hyperuricemia, hypercholesterolemia, hypertriglyceridemia, and the so-called atherogenic dyslipidemia (i.e., low levels of high-density lipoprotein [HDL] cholesterol and high levels of triglycerides). It should be also noted that these alterations may have reciprocal interactions with hypertension. In fact, from one side they can be induced by hypertension, and from the other side they may promote sustained increase of blood pressure levels. In addition, it has been recently reported that several antihypertensive drug classes or molecules may induce glucose and lipid impairments, thus promoting the new onset of either diabetes or dyslipidemia, which of course has negative prognostic impact on the natural history of hypertension and hypertension-related major cardiovascular complications. Thus, the presence of hypertension should always stimulate a thorough assessment of the individual metabolic profile, which contributes to properly define individual global cardiovascular risk profile

For these reasons, and in view of the increasing prevalence in the general population of hypertensive patients, closer attention should be devoted to effective prevention, early identification, and prompt treatment of different metabolic abnormalities that can be associated with hypertension. Indeed, current international guidelines clearly identify some specific antihypertensive drug classes that should be preferred when treating hypertensive patients with metabolic abnormalities.

In this volume of *Practical Case Studies in Hypertension Management*, the clinical management of paradigmatic cases of patients with hypertension and metabolic abnormalities will be discussed, focusing on the different diagnostic criteria currently available for identifying the presence of these metabolic impairments, as well as on the different therapeutic options to be used for achieving effective and sustained blood pressure control and reducing the potential drug-related side effects or adverse metabolic reactions to various antihypertensive drug classes.

Rome, Italy

Giuliano Tocci
Editor of the Series

Contents

1 Clinical Case 1: Patient with Essential Hypertension and Metabolic Syndrome 1
1.1 Clinical Case Presentation 1
Family History 1
Clinical History 2
Physical Examination 2
Haematological Profile 3
Blood Pressure Profile 3
12-Lead Electrocardiogram 4
Current Treatment 4
Diagnosis 4
Global Cardiovascular Risk Stratification 5
Treatment Evaluation 6
Prescriptions 6
1.2 Follow-Up (Visit 1) at 6 Weeks 6
Physical Examination 6
Blood Pressure Profile 7
Current Treatment 7
Diagnostic Tests for Organ Damage or Associated Clinical Conditions 7
Diagnosis 8
Global Cardiovascular Risk Stratification 8
Treatment Evaluation 9
Prescriptions 9
1.3 Follow-Up (Visit 2) at 3 Months 9
Physical Examination 9
Blood Pressure Profile 9
Current Treatment 10
Treatment Evaluation 10

Prescriptions 10
1.4 Follow-Up (Visit 3) at 1 Year 10
Physical Examination 10
Haematological Profile 11
Blood Pressure Profile 11
Diagnostic Tests for Organ Damage or Associated Clinical Conditions 11
Current Treatment 11
Treatment Evaluation 12
Prescriptions 12
1.5 Discussion 13
References 15

2 Clinical Case 2: Adult Patient with Hypertension and Diabetes 17
2.1 Clinical Case Presentation 17
Family History 17
Clinical History 18
Physical Examination 18
Haematological Profile 18
Blood Pressure Profile 19
12-Lead Electrocardiogram 19
Current Treatment 20
Diagnosis 21
Global Cardiovascular Risk Stratification 21
Treatment Evaluation 21
Prescriptions 22
2.2 Follow-Up (Visit 1) at 6 Weeks 22
Physical Examination 22
Blood Pressure Profile 22
Current Treatment 22
Diagnostic Tests for Organ Damage or Associated Clinical Conditions 23
Diagnosis 23
Global Cardiovascular Risk Stratification 24
Treatment Evaluation 24
Prescriptions 25
2.3 Follow-Up (Visit 2) at 3 Months 25
Physical Examination 25

Blood Pressure Profile 25
Haematological Profile 25
Current Treatment 26
Treatment Evaluation 26
Prescriptions 26
2.4 Follow-Up (Visit 3) at 1 Year 26
Physical Examination 26
Haematological Profile 27
Blood Pressure Profile 27
Diagnostic Tests for Organ Damage or Associated Clinical Conditions 28
Current Treatment 28
Treatment Evaluation 28
Prescriptions 29
2.5 Discussion 29
References 31

3 Clinical Case 3: Patient with Essential Hypertension and Familial Hypercholesterolaemia 33
3.1 Clinical Case Presentation 33
Family History 33
Clinical History 34
Physical Examination 34
Haematological Profile 34
Blood Pressure Profile 36
Twelve-Lead Electrocardiogram 36
Current Treatment 36
Diagnosis 37
Global Cardiovascular Risk Stratification 37
Treatment Evaluation 39
Prescriptions 39
3.2 Follow-Up (Visit 1) at 6 Weeks 39
Physical Examination 40
Blood Pressure Profile 40
Current Treatment 41
Diagnostic Tests for Organ Damage or Associated Clinical Conditions 41
Diagnosis 42

Global Cardiovascular Risk Stratification 42
Treatment Evaluation 43
Prescriptions 43
3.3 Follow-Up (Visit 2) at 3 Months 43
Physical Examination 43
Blood Pressure Profile 43
Current Treatment 43
Treatment Evaluation 44
Prescriptions 44
3.4 Follow-Up (Visit 3) at 1 Year 44
Physical Examination 44
Haematological Profile 44
Blood Pressure Profile 45
Diagnostic Tests for Organ Damage
or Associated Clinical Conditions 46
Current Treatment 46
Treatment Evaluation 46
Prescriptions 46
3.5 Discussion 47
References 49

4 Clinical Case 4: Patient with Essential Hypertension and Hypertriglyceridaemia 51
4.1 Clinical Case Presentation 51
Family History 51
Clinical History 52
Physical Examination 52
Haematological Profile 52
Blood Pressure Profile 53
Twelve-Lead Electrocardiogram 53
Current Treatment 54
Diagnosis 54
Global Cardiovascular Risk Stratification 55
Treatment Evaluation 55
Prescriptions 56
4.2 Follow-Up (Visit 1) at 6 Weeks 56
Physical Examination 56
Blood Pressure Profile 56
Current Treatment 57

Diagnostic Tests for Organ Damage or Associated Clinical Conditions 57
Diagnosis 57
Global Cardiovascular Risk Stratification 58
Treatment Evaluation 59
Prescriptions 60
4.3 Follow-Up (Visit 2) at 3 Months 60
Physical Examination 60
Blood Pressure Profile 60
Haematological Profile 60
Current Treatment 61
Treatment Evaluation 61
Prescriptions 61
4.4 Follow-Up (Visit 3) at 1 Year 61
Physical Examination 61
Haematological Profile 62
Blood Pressure Profile 62
Diagnostic Tests for Organ Damage or Associated Clinical Conditions 63
Current Treatment 63
Treatment Evaluation Current Treatment 63
Prescriptions 63
4.5 Discussion 64
References 66

5 Clinical Case 5: Patient with Essential Hypertension and Moderate Obesity 69
5.1 Clinical Case Presentation 69
Family History 69
Clinical History 70
Physical Examination 70
Haematological Profile 70
Blood Pressure Profile 71
Twelve-Lead Electrocardiogram 71
Current Treatment 72
Diagnosis 72
Global Cardiovascular Risk Stratification 73
Treatment Evaluation 73
Prescriptions 74

5.2 Follow-Up (Visit 1) at 6 Weeks 74
Physical Examination 74
Blood Pressure Profile 74
Current Treatment. 74
Diagnostic Tests for Organ Damage
or Associated Clinical Conditions. 75
Diagnosis 75
Global Cardiovascular Risk Stratification 75
Treatment Evaluation. 76
Prescriptions 76
5.3 Follow-Up (Visit 2) at 3 Months. 76
Physical Examination 76
Blood Pressure Profile 77
Current Treatment. 77
Treatment Evaluation. 77
Prescriptions 77
5.4 Follow-Up (Visit 3) at 1 Year 77
Physical Examination 78
Haematological Profile. 78
Blood Pressure Profile 78
Diagnostic Tests for Organ Damage
or Associated Clinical Conditions. 79
Current Treatment. 79
Treatment Evaluation. 79
Prescriptions 80
5.5 Discussion 80
References. 82

**6 Clinical Case 6: Adult Patient
with Hypertension and Gout** 85
6.1 Clinical Case Presentation. 85
Family History 85
Clinical History 86
Physical Examination 86
Haematological Profile. 86
Blood Pressure Profile 87
Twelve-Lead Electrocardiogram. 87
Current Treatment. 88
Diagnosis 88

Global Cardiovascular Risk Stratification 89
Treatment Evaluation 90
Prescriptions 90
6.2 Follow-Up (Visit 1) at 6 Weeks 90
Physical Examination 91
Blood Pressure Profile 91
Current Treatment 91
Diagnostic Tests for Organ Damage
or Associated Clinical Conditions 91
Diagnosis 91
Global Cardiovascular Risk Stratification 92
Treatment Evaluation 93
Prescriptions 93
6.3 Follow-Up (Visit 2) at 3 Months 93
Physical Examination 94
Blood Pressure Profile 94
Haematological Profile 94
Current Treatment 94
Treatment Evaluation 95
Prescriptions 95
6.4 Follow-Up (Visit 3) at 1 Year 95
Physical Examination 95
Haematological Profile 96
Blood Pressure Profile 96
Diagnostic Tests for Organ Damage
or Associated Clinical Conditions 96
Current Treatment 98
Treatment Evaluation 99
Prescriptions 99
6.5 Discussion 99
References 101

Chapter 1
Clinical Case 1: Patient with Essential Hypertension and Metabolic Syndrome

1.1 Clinical Case Presentation

Man, 70 years old, ex-smoker since 10 years (20 smoked cigarettes for 30 years), and overweight after the retirement (10 years ago), when his blood pressure began to increase. Eight years ago, he began to take atenolol 50 mg in the morning, and then it was interrupted because of bradycardia. Therefore, 4 years ago he began taking ramipril/hydrochlorothiazide 5/25 mg ½ tablet each morning. Lately, his general practitioner (GP) added doxazosin 2 mg 1 tablet taken at 2 o'clock in the afternoon, because of suboptimal BP control. He usually does not care much about his health, but he comes to our hypertension clinic for a general checkup, hoping to reduce the number of tablets he takes each day.

Family History

The father of the patient died because of sudden death (no autopsy executed) at the age of 68, being affected by type 2 diabetes from the age of 57. His mother is yet living, 94 y.o.,

A.F.G. Cicero, *Hypertension and Metabolic Cardiovascular Risk Factors*, Practical Case Studies in Hypertension Management, DOI 10.1007/978-3-319-39504-3_1,

overweight, but not hypertensive nor diabetic. He has a younger brother, 68 y.o., affected by stable angina from the age of 45 and liver cirrhosis, with an old history of heavy smoking habit (40 cigarettes/day), sedentariness, and heavy alcohol consumption (not less than 1 l of wine and 2–3 shots per day).

Clinical History

The patient has a relatively long list of cardiovascular risk factors: high blood pressure, atherogenic dyslipidaemia, impaired fasting glucose, ECG signs of left ventricular hypertrophy, and mild microalbuminuria, but no history of cardio- and cerebrovascular events. Overweight and sedentary lifestyle also contribute to the cardiovascular risk profile of the patient, even if they are not included among the risk factors considered in the risk stratification following the ESH/ESC guidelines.

Physical Examination

- Weight: 78.2 kg.
- Height: 1.71 cm.
- Body mass index (BMI): 27.7 kg/m^2.
- Waist circumference: 103 cm.
- Respiration: auscultation of the chest reveals clear lung fields and no murmurs or rubs.
- Heart sounds: regular rhythm, no accessory murmurs.
- Resting pulse: regular, 72 bpm.
- Carotid arteries: no bruit on auscultation.
- Femoral and foot arteries: all pulses present and normosphygmic.
- Abdomen: moderately globular, liver inferior border palpable 2 cm below the costal margin.

Haematological Profile

- Haemoglobin: 14.1 g/dL
- Haematocrit: 43 %
- Fasting plasma glucose: 112 mg/dL
- Fasting lipids: total cholesterol (TOT-C), 198 mg/dl; low-density lipoprotein cholesterol (LDL-C), 83 mg/dl; high-density lipoprotein cholesterol (HDL-C), 39 mg/dl; triglycerides (TG) 382 mg/dl
- Electrolytes: sodium, 139 mEq/L; potassium, 3.8 mEq/L
- Serum uric acid: 5.5 mg/dL
- Renal function: urea, 25 mg/dl; creatinine, 1.0 mg/dL; creatinine clearance (Cockroft-Gault), 75.8 ml/min; estimated glomerular filtration rate (eGFR) (MDRD), 78.5 mL/min/1.73 m^2
- Urine analysis (dipstick): gravity 1020, pH 6.8, no glucose nor sediments
- Albuminuria: 42 mg/24 h
- Liver function tests: GOT, 30 U/L; GPT, 38 U/L; gamma-GT, 54 mg/dL (suggestive of a nonalcoholic fatty liver disease)
- Thyroid function tests: in the normal range

Blood Pressure Profile

- Home BP (average): 150/78 mmHg
- Sitting BP: 158/79 mmHg (right arm); 160/78 mmHg (left arm)
- Standing BP: 156/78 mmHg at 1 min
- 24 h BP: 148/82 mmHg; HR, 71 bpm
- Daytime BP: 153/85 mmHg; HR, 74 bpm
- Night-time BP: 136/77 mmHg; HR, 65 bpm

24 h ambulatory blood pressure profile is illustrated in Fig. 1.1.

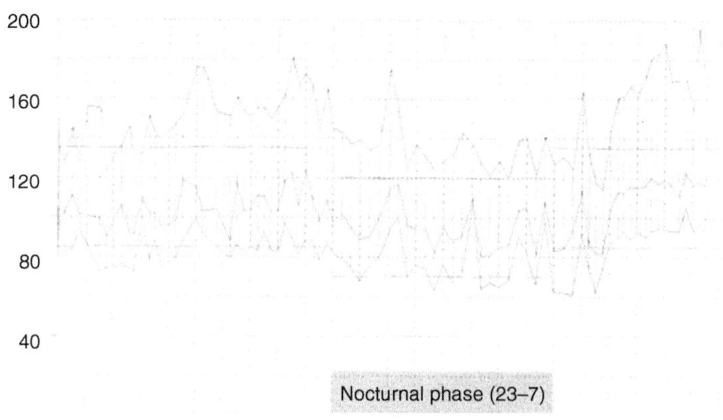

FIGURE 1.1 Baseline patient 24-h ambulatory blood pressure chart

12-Lead Electrocardiogram

The standard 12-lead ECG show signs of left ventricular hypertrophy (Fig. 1.2).

Current Treatment

- Ramipril/hydrochlorothiazide 5/25 mg ½ tablet h. 8.00
- Doxazosin 2 mg 1 tablet h. 14.00
- ASA 100 mg 1 tablet after lunch
- Atorvastatin 10 mg 1 tablet h. 22.00

Diagnosis

Grade I hypertension in metabolic syndrome diagnosed following the last internationally harmonized diagnostic criteria (5 criteria on 5!) [1], complicated by electrocardiographically diagnosed left ventricular hypertrophy and microalbuminuria.

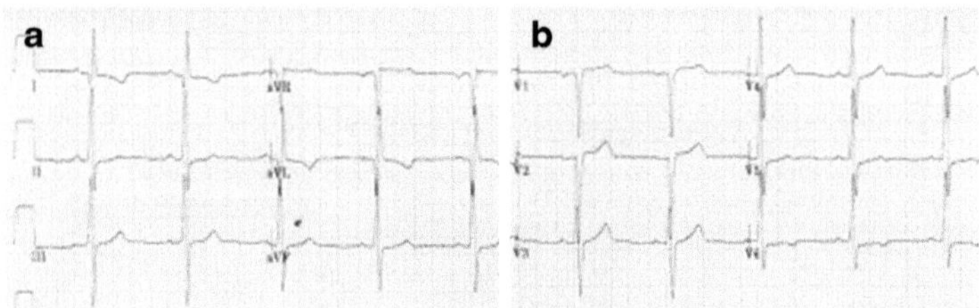

FIGURE 1.2 (**a**, **b**). Patient baseline standard 12-lead ECG. Left ventricular hypertrophy with Sokolow index=37 mm, mild ST depression in V1 and V2, negative T waves in D1, aVL, V6

In the light of the available information, what is the estimated cardiovascular risk of the patient?

Possible answers are:

1. Low
2. Medium
3. High
4. Very high

Global Cardiovascular Risk Stratification

The patient has more than two additional risk factors but also left ventricular hypertrophy and microalbuminuria; therefore he has to be classified as a subject with high added cardiovascular risk [2].

Which is the best therapeutic option for this patient at this step?

Possible answers are:

1. Add another drug class (e.g. dihydropyridinic calcium antagonist).
2. Add another drug class (e.g. beta-blocker).
3. Increase the diuretic dose.

4. Switch from the association of an ACE inhibitor with thiazides to ACE inhibitor with calcium antagonist adequately dosed.
5. Switch from ACE inhibitor to direct renin inhibitor combined with thiazide diuretic.

Treatment Evaluation

- Ramipril 5/25 mg ½ tablet and doxazosin 2 mg changed with ramipril 10 mg/amlodipine 5 mg in 1 tablet h. 8.00
- ASA 100 mg 1 tablet after lunch (unchanged)
- Atorvastatin 10 mg 1 tablet h. 22.00 (unchanged)

Prescriptions

- Therapeutic lifestyle prescription, in particular the patient was instructed to follow general indications of a Mediterranean diet, avoiding excessive intake of dairy products and red meat, increasing the intake of vegetables, and reducing as possible the consumption of salt. Moreover, he was also encouraged to increase his physical activity by walking briskly for 20 to 30 min, three to five times per week, or by cycling.
- Carotid echo-colour Doppler examination.

1.2 Follow-Up (Visit 1) at 6 Weeks

The patient is satisfied with the reduction of tablet number to be taken in a day and claims that his BP at home is "perfectly controlled". He states to have put stronger attention to his diet, significantly reducing the content of salt and total energy, but not to have really improved the weekly physical activity.

Physical Examination

- Overall unchanged, when compared with the previous visit. The patient lost 0.6 kg.

Blood Pressure Profile

- Home BP (average): 143/76 mmHg
- Sitting BP: 149/80 mmHg
- Standing BP: 148/78 mmHg

Current Treatment

- Therapeutic lifestyle
- Ramipril 10 mg/amlodipine 5 mg in 1 tablet h. 8.00
- ASA 100 mg 1 tablet after lunch
- Atorvastatin 10 mg 1 tablet h. 22.00

Diagnostic Tests for Organ Damage or Associated Clinical Conditions

The carotid echo-colour Doppler ultrasound examination shows irregular plaques at both bulbs, with a bilateral stenosis of 40–45 % without significant haemodynamic effects (Fig. 1.3).

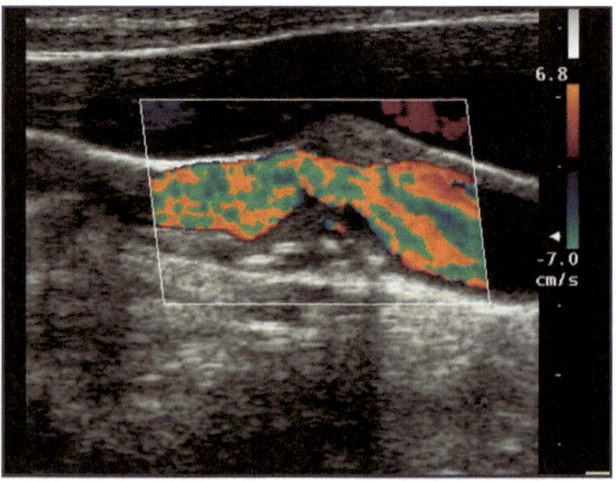

Figure 1.3 Patient carotid Doppler ultrasound

Diagnosis

Grade I hypertension in metabolic syndrome diagnosed following the ATP III criteria (5 criteria on 5!), complicated by electrocardiographically diagnosed left ventricular hypertrophy, carotid plaques, and microalbuminuria.

In the light of the available information, what is the estimated cardiovascular risk of the patient?

Possible answers are:

1. Low
2. Medium
3. High
4. Very high

Global Cardiovascular Risk Stratification

Despite BP control improvement, the patient has more than two additional risk factors but also left ventricular hypertrophy and microalbuminuria, so that he has to be classified as a subject with high added cardiovascular risk [2].

Which is the best therapeutic option for this patient at this step?

Possible answers are:

1. Add another drug class (e.g. alpha-agonist).
2. Add another drug class (e.g. beta-blocker).
3. Add another drug class (e.g. diuretic).
4. Increase the calcium antagonist dose.
5. Switch from ACE inhibitor to direct renin inhibitor.

Treatment Evaluation

- Therapeutic lifestyle
- Ramipril 10 mg/amlodipine 10 mg in 1 tablet h. 8.00 (amlodipine dosage doubled)
- ASA 100 mg 1 tablet after lunch
- Atorvastatin 20 mg 1 tablet h. 22.00 (Atorvastatin dosage doubled)

Prescriptions

- Intensification of therapeutic lifestyle measures, with particular attention to physical activity
- Lipid pattern with liver transaminases, gamma-GT, and CPK

1.3 Follow-Up (Visit 2) at 3 Months

The patient reports further improvement in home BP values without subjective side effects. He continues to care about diet, and he began to practise some physical activity (even if not so intensively as prescribed).

Physical Examination

- Body weight decreased 3 kg from the first visit.
- No changes as it regards other apparati.

Blood Pressure Profile

- Home BP (average): 139/76 mmHg
- Sitting BP: 141/78 mmHg
- Standing BP: 138/76 mmHg

Current Treatment

- Ramipril 10 mg/amlodipine 10 mg in 1 tablet h. 8.00
- ASA 100 mg 1 tablet after lunch
- Atorvastatin 20 mg 1 tablet h. 22.00

Treatment Evaluation

- No drug has been modified.
- No drug dose has been changed.

Prescriptions

- Maintenance of therapeutic lifestyle measures
- Full haematochemistry and urinalysis

1.4 Follow-Up (Visit 3) at 1 Year

The patient reports a good adherence to the prescribed therapy and to the therapeutic lifestyle changes. He lost more weight. The glucose, lipid, and liver parameters strongly improved until normalization, with further improvement in home BP values without subjective side effects.

Physical Examination

- Weight: 70.9 kg
- Height: 1.71 cm
- Body mass index (BMI): 24.3 kg/m^2
- Waist circumference: 95 cm
- Abdomen: normal, liver inferior border no more palpable below the costal margin

Haematological Profile

- Fasting plasma glucose: 99 mg/dL
- Fasting lipids: total cholesterol (TOT-C), 162 mg/dl; low-density lipoprotein cholesterol (LDL-C), 76 mg/dl; high-density lipoprotein cholesterol (HDL-C), 46 mg/dl; triglycerides (TG), 199 mg/dl
- Liver function tests: GOT 21 U/L, GPT 26 U/L, gamma-GT 38 mg/dL
- CPK = 174 U/L

Blood Pressure Profile

- Home BP (average): 130/76 mmHg
- Sitting BP: 136/78 mmHg (right arm); 135/76 mmHg (left arm)
- Standing BP: 134/77 mmHg at 1 min
- 24-h BP: 124/74 mmHg; HR: 67 bpm
- Daytime BP: 127/78 mmHg; HR: 70 bpm
- Night-time BP: 110/65 mmHg; HR: 63 bpm

24 h ambulatory blood pressure profile is illustrated in Fig. 1.4.

Diagnostic Tests for Organ Damage or Associated Clinical Conditions

Albuminuria decreased in the normal range (22 mg/24 h); however the risk of the patient remains high because of the permanence of other signs of target organ damage (carotid plaques, left ventricular hypertrophy)

Current Treatment

- Therapeutic lifestyle

- Ramipril 10 mg/amlodipine 10 mg in 1 tablet h. 8.00
- ASA 100 mg 1 tablet after lunch
- Atorvastatin 20 mg 1 tablet h. 22.00

Treatment Evaluation

- Therapeutic lifestyle (confirmed)
- Ramipril 10 mg/amlodipine 10 mg in 1 tablet h. 8.00 (confirmed)
- ASA 100 mg 1 tablet after lunch (confirmed)
- Atorvastatin 20 mg 1 tablet h. 22.00 (confirmed)

Prescriptions

- Periodical BP evaluation at home according to recommendations from current guidelines.
- Standard 12-ECG once a year
- Carotid ultrasound once a year

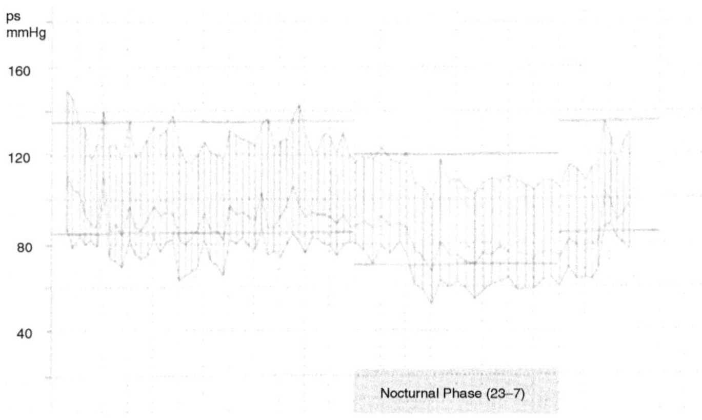

FIGURE 1.4 Patient post-treatment 24-h ambulatory blood pressure chart

Which will be the most useful diagnostic test to repeat during the follow-up in this patient?

Possible answers are:

1. Electrocardiogram
2. Echocardiogram
3. Vascular Doppler ultrasound
4. Evaluation of renal parameters (e.g. creatininaemia, eGFR, ClCr, UACR)
5. Twenty-four-hour ambulatory BP monitoring

1.5 Discussion

The metabolic syndrome is a complex multifactorial disease associated with increased risk of cardiovascular diseases, type 2 diabetes, and all-cause mortality. Its prevalence is about 30 % in general adult population and includes, as a main component of its definition, hypertension, which could appear before the development of a full metabolic syndrome or like a consequence of a pre-existing insulin resistance and overweight [3]. The possible genetic predisposition and the lifestyle of the patients affected by metabolic syndrome strongly influence the severity of the syndrome and the answer to drug treatment [4] (Fig. 1.5).

The clinical case here described is prototypical. The patient did not care about his health until the complete checkup. Therefore, when he clearly understood to be at risk to develop cardiovascular diseases and type 2 diabetes, with an adequate education, he has improved his lifestyle and, consequently, the level of risk parameters strongly related to cardiovascular risk: hypertension, impaired fasting glucose, hypertriglyceridaemia, and low plasma HDL cholesterol level.

On the other side, both the antihypertensive and lipid-lowering drugs had to be improved in order to obtain an optimization of both BP and LDL-C levels.

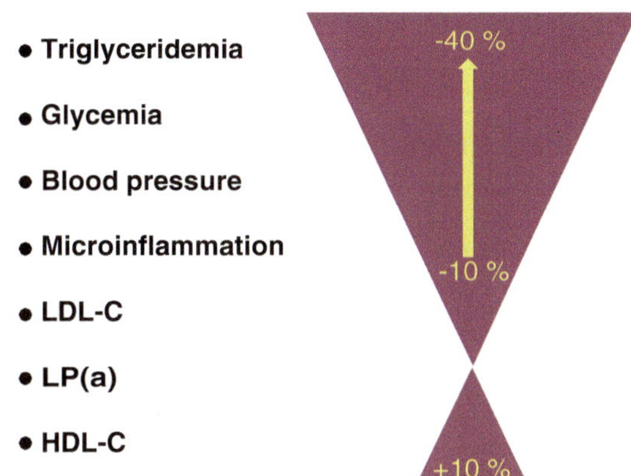

FIGURE 1.5 Relative efficacy of lifestyle change in improving different metabolic syndrome components (and related cardiovascular risk factors) (Personal unpublished figure)

Regarding the choice of the antihypertensive treatment, in this kind of patients, the guidelines suggest to prefer metabolically neutral drugs, like renin-angiotensin-aldosterone system blocking drug and/or calcium antagonists, maintaining thiazides or beta-blockers as second choices, when not strictly required [2]. A combined treatment has been chosen in order to improve the ability (and the will) of the patient to regularly take his daily therapy [5].

Statin dose was also doubled in order to reach a more strict LDL-C control in the context of a global improvement of cardiovascular risk [6]. This patient reminds the ones enrolled in the large Anglo-Scandinavian Cardiac Outcomes Trial—Lipid Lowering Arm (ASCOT-LLA) trial, where the combination of amlodipine and atorvastatin consented to reach the most significant reduction in cardiovascular disease risk [7].

Of course, the management of the patient was not totally based on guidelines. For instance, the guidelines would have suggested to increase drug dosages or number to optimize both blood pressure and atherogenic dyslipidaemia from the second visit. However, the patient seemed to be keen to modify his lifestyle, while BP was just significantly improved, so we decided to test the ability of the patient to more strictly follow the suggested therapeutic lifestyle indications. The results obtained on the next visit prised our confidence in the patient will.

Take-Home Messages

- Metabolic syndrome is highly prevalent in general population and hypertension is the most frequent component of the syndrome.
- The overlapping of metabolic syndrome with hypertension strongly increases the risk to develop hypertension-related complication (in particular cardiovascular events).
- No drug specifically improves metabolic syndrome, but therapeutic lifestyle can significantly improve both metabolic syndrome and blood pressure control.
- When treating metabolic syndrome patients, it is relevant to choose antihypertensive drugs without metabolic interference with glucose and lipid metabolism.
- Blockers of the renin-angiotensin-aldosterone system and calcium antagonists are usually preferred for the management of hypertensive patients with metabolic syndrome.

References

1. Alberti KG, Eckel RH, Grundy SM, Zimmet PZ, Cleeman JI, Donato KA, Fruchart JC, James WP, Loria CM, Smith Jr SC. Harmonizing the metabolic syndrome: a joint interim statement of the International Diabetes Federation Task Force on Epidemiology and Prevention; National Heart, Lung, and Blood Institute; American Heart Association; World Heart Federation; International Atherosclerosis Society; and International Association for the Study of Obesity. Circulation. 2009;120:1640–5.
2. Mancia G, Fagard R, Narkiewicz K, Redon J, Zanchetti A, Bohm M, et al. 2013 ESH/ESC Guidelines for the management of arte-

rial hypertension: the Task Force for the management of arterial hypertension of the European Society of Hypertension (ESH) and of the European Society of Cardiology (ESC). J Hypertens. 2013;31(7):1281–357.

3. Grundy SM. Metabolic syndrome update. Trends Cardiovasc Med. 2015;pii:S1050-1738(15)00249-2.
4. Takahara M, Shimomura I. Metabolic syndrome and lifestyle modification. Rev Endocr Metab Disord. 2014;15(4):317–27.
5. Olszanecka-Glinianowicz M, Smertka M, Almgren-Rachtan A, Chudek J. Ramipril/amlodipine single pill – effectiveness, tolerance and patient satisfaction with antihypertensive therapy in relation to nutritional status. Pharmacol Rep. 2014;66(6):1043–9.
6. European Association for Cardiovascular Prevention & Rehabilitation, Reiner Z, Catapano AL, De Backer G, Graham I, Taskinen MR, Wiklund O, Agewall S, Alegria E, Chapman MJ, Durrington P, Erdine S, Halcox J, Hobbs R, Kjekshus J, Filardi PP, Riccardi G, Storey RF, Wood D, ESC Committee for Practice Guidelines (CPG) 2008–2010 and 2010–2012 Committees. ESC/EAS Guidelines for the management of dyslipidaemias: the Task Force for the management of dyslipidaemias of the European Society of Cardiology (ESC) and the European Atherosclerosis Society (EAS). Eur Heart J. 2011;32(14):1769–818.
7. Sever P, Dahlöf B, Poulter N, Wedel H, Beevers G, Caulfield M, Collins R, Kjeldsen S, Kristinsson A, McInnes G, Mehlsen J, Nieminem M, O'Brien E, Ostergren J, ASCOT Steering Committee Members. Potential synergy between lipid-lowering and blood-pressure-lowering in the Anglo-Scandinavian Cardiac Outcomes Trial. Eur Heart J. 2006;27(24):2982–8.

Chapter 2
Clinical Case 2: Adult Patient with Hypertension and Diabetes

2.1 Clinical Case Presentation

Woman, 64 years old, occasional smoker at a young age (4–5 smoked cigarettes per week for 10 years), overweight since menopause (at the age of 51) and her blood pressure began to increase. Seven years ago, she was discovered to be affected by type 2 diabetes, initially controlled with diet only and then treated with metformin and glibenclamide. Initially, her hypertension was treated with enalapril 20 mg, but lately her GP added hydrochlorothiazide 25 mg 1 tablet taken at 12 noon, because of suboptimal BP control. The patient is really worried for her health, fearing about the possible long-term effects of high blood pressure and type 2 diabetes on her survival.

Family History

The patient's mother died at the age of 73 because of type 2 diabetes complications (blind, demented, and with peripheral occlusive artery disease). Her younger brother (59 years old) is also diabetic and hypertensive. Her son, 42 years old, is overweight and has metabolic syndrome, with borderline blood pressure values and impaired fasting glucose.

A.F.G. Cicero, *Hypertension and Metabolic Cardiovascular Risk Factors*, Practical Case Studies in Hypertension Management, DOI 10.1007/978-3-319-39504-3_2,

Clinical History

The patient's history is relatively ordinary for an overweight, diabetic, and hypertensive subject. However, during the last period (5–6 months), she has diurnal tiredness and perceives a disturbed sleep, even if her husband states that she sleeps regularly without snoring nor awakenings. Sometimes, the tiredness appears suddenly and she feels to pass out. She is not sure if this could be related to blood pressure or glucose rapid changes, since usually she recovers in a couple of minutes and then she does not care about it.

Physical Examination

- Weight: 79.3 kg.
- Height: 1.69 cm.
- Body mass index (BMI): 27.7 kg/m^2.
- Waist circumference: 95 cm.
- Respiration: auscultation of the chest reveals clear lung fields and no murmurs or rubs.
- Heart sounds: regular rhythm, no accessory murmurs.
- Resting pulse: regular, 78 bpm.
- Carotid arteries: no bruit on auscultation.
- Femoral and foot arteries: all pulses present, but mildly attenuated at the pretibial level.
- Abdomen: moderately globular, inferior margin of liver not palpable.

Haematological Profile

- Haemoglobin: 13.9 g/dL
- Haematocrit: 44 %
- Fasting plasma glucose: 153 mg/dL
- Glycated haemoglobin (HbA1c): 61 mmol/mol (7.7 %)

- Fasting lipids: total cholesterol (TOT-C), 191 mg/dl; low-density lipoprotein cholesterol (LDL-C), 112 mg/dl; high-density lipoprotein cholesterol (HDL-C), 42 mg/dl; triglycerides (TG), 185 mg/dl
- Electrolytes: sodium, 140 mEq/L; potassium, 3.9 mEq/L
- Serum uric acid: 5.7 mg/dL
- Renal function: urea, 27 mg/dl; creatinine, 0.8 mg/dL; creatinine clearance (Cockroft-Gault), 88.9 ml/min; estimated glomerular filtration rate (eGFR) (MDRD), 72 mL/min/1.73 m^2
- Urine analysis (dipstick): gravity 1025, pH 6.5, no glucose nor sediments
- Albuminuria: 13 mg/24 h
- Liver function tests: GOT, 24 U/L; GPT, 27 U/L; gamma-GT, 31 mg/dL
- Thyroid function tests: in the normal range

Blood Pressure Profile

- Home BP (average): 135/74 mmHg
- Sitting BP: 138/80 mmHg (right arm); 136/78 mmHg (left arm)
- Standing BP: 136/76 mmHg at 1 min
- 24 h BP: 134/74 mmHg; HR: 70 bpm
- Daytime BP: 133/75 mmHg; HR, 75 bpm
- Night-time BP: 137/70 mmHg; HR, 54 bpm

24 h ambulatory blood pressure profile is illustrated in Fig. 2.1.

12-Lead Electrocardiogram

The standard 12-lead ECG show signs of an incomplete right branch bundle block with an RSR' pattern in V1-3 with QRS duration < 120 m/s (Fig. 2.2).

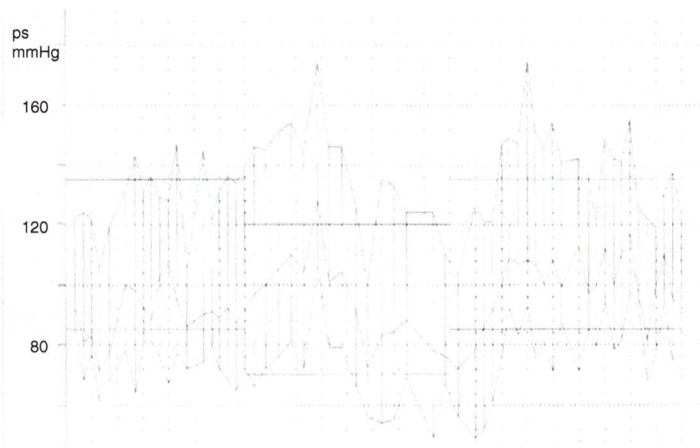

FIGURE 2.1 Baseline patient 24-h ambulatory blood pressure chart

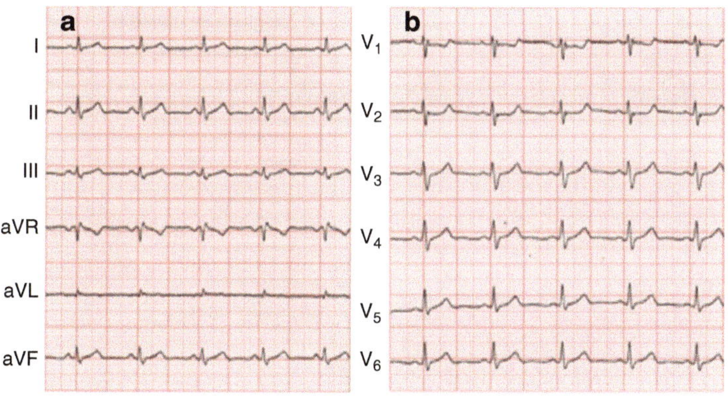

FIGURE 2.2 (**a**, **b**). Patient baseline standard 12-lead ECG

Current Treatment

- Enalapril 20 mg 1 tablet h. 8.00
- Hydrochlorothiazide 25 mg 1 tablet h. 14.00
- Metformin 500 mg 1 tablet h. 12.00 and 1 tablet h. 20.00
- Glibenclamide 5 mg 1 tablet h. 12.00

- ASA 100 mg 1 tablet after lunch
- Atorvastatin 20 mg 1 tablet h. 22.00

Diagnosis

High normal blood pressure values under antihypertensive treatment [1], in suboptimally controlled type 2 diabetes and overweight.

In the light of the available information, what is the estimated cardiovascular risk of the patient?

Possible answers are:

1. Low
2. Medium
3. High
4. Very high

Global Cardiovascular Risk Stratification

Even if the blood pressure control is relatively good, the presence of type 2 diabetes makes the patient be classified as a subject with (at least) moderate to high added cardiovascular risk [1].

Treatment Evaluation

- Enalapril/lercanidipine 20/20 mg 1 tablet h. 8.00 (modified by substituting, in the same tablet, diuretics with lercanidipine)
- Metformin/sitagliptin 850/50 mg 1 tablet h. 8.00 and 1 tablet h. 20.00 (modified by substituting, in the same tablet, glibenclamide with sitagliptin and mildly increasing metformin dosage)
- ASA 100 mg 1 tablet after lunch (unchanged)
- Atorvastatin 20 mg 1 tablet h. 22.00 (unchanged)

Prescriptions

- Therapeutic lifestyle prescription, in particular the patient was instructed to follow the general indications of a Mediterranean diet, avoiding excessive intake of dairy products and red meat, increasing the intake of vegetables, and reducing as possible the consumption of salt. Moreover, he was also encouraged to increase her physical activity by walking briskly for 20 to 30 min, three to five times per week, or by cycling.
- Carotid echo-colour Doppler examination.

2.2 Follow-Up (Visit 1) at 6 Weeks

The patient is satisfied with the reduction of tablet number to be taken daily and claims that she has no more episodes of sudden weakness. She states to have put stronger attention to her diet, significantly reducing the content of salt and total energy, but not to have improved the weekly physical activity.

Physical Examination

- Overall unchanged, when compared with the previous visit. The patient lost 1.0 kg.

Blood Pressure Profile

- Home BP (average): 136/75 mmHg
- Sitting BP: 138/80 mmHg
- Standing BP: 135/76 mmHg

Current Treatment

- Enalapril/lercanidipine 20/20 mg 1 tablet h. 8.00
- Metformin/sitagliptin 850/50 mg 1 tablet h. 8.00 and 1 tablet h. 20.00

- ASA 100 mg 1 tablet after lunch
- Atorvastatin 20 mg 1 tablet h. 22.00

Diagnostic Tests for Organ Damage or Associated Clinical Conditions

The carotid echo-colour Doppler ultrasound examination shows irregular plaques at both bulbs, with a bilateral stenosis of 45–50 % in absence of significant haemodynamic effects (Fig. 2.3).

Diagnosis

High normal blood pressure values under antihypertensive treatment [1], in suboptimally controlled type 2 diabetes and overweight, complicated by carotid atherosclerosis.

In the light of the available information, what is the estimated cardiovascular risk of the patient?

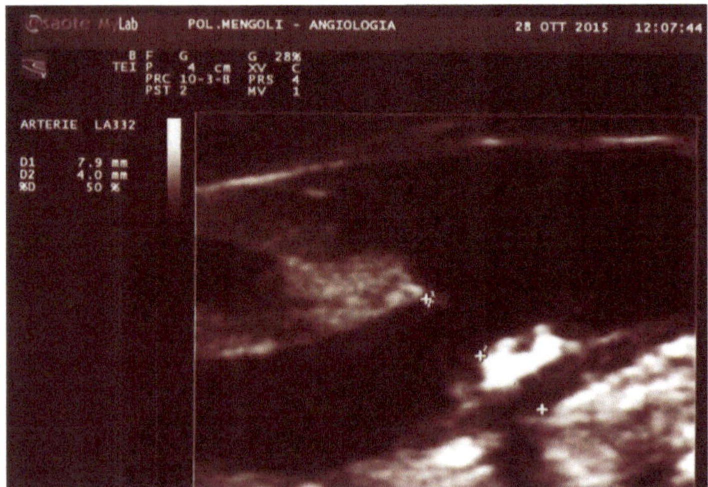

FIGURE 2.3 Patient carotid Doppler ultrasound

Possible answers are:

1. Low
2. Medium
3. High
4. Very high

Global Cardiovascular Risk Stratification

With the discovery of carotid atherosclerosis, associated with the diagnosis of type 2 diabetes, the patient's added cardiovascular risk has to be reclassified to very high [1].

Which is the best therapeutic option for this patient at this step?

Possible answers are:

1. Add another antihypertensive drug class (e.g. dihydropyridinic calcium antagonist).
2. Add another antihypertensive drug class (e.g. beta-blocker).
3. Strengthen lifestyle suggestion and add another lipid-lowering drug (e.g. ezetimibe).
4. Switch from ACE inhibitor to direct renin inhibitor.

Treatment Evaluation

- Therapeutic lifestyle
- Enalapril/lercanidipine 20/20 mg 1 tablet h. 8.00 (unchanged)
- Metformin/sitagliptin 850/50 mg 1 tablet h. 8.00 and 1 tablet h. 20.00 (unchanged)
- ASA 100 mg 1 tablet after lunch (unchanged)
- Atorvastatin 20 mg 1 tablet h. 22.00 (unchanged)
- Ezetimibe 10 mg 1 tablet h. 22.00 (added)

Prescriptions

- Intensification of the therapeutic lifestyle measures, with particular attention to physical activity
- Fasting plasma glucose, glycated haemoglobin, lipid pattern with liver transaminases, gamma-GT, and CPK

2.3 Follow-Up (Visit 2) at 3 Months

The patient reports to feel fine. She continues to care about diet and she began a training program with a personal trainer in a specialized sport centre.

Physical Examination

- Body weight decreased 3.5 kg since the first visit.
- No changes as it regards others apparati.

Blood Pressure Profile

- Home BP (average): 134/76 mmHg
- Sitting BP: 136/78 mmHg
- Standing BP: 136/75 mmHg

Haematological Profile

- Fasting plasma glucose: 124 mg/dL
- Glycated haemoglobin (HbA1c): 54 mmol/mol (7.1 %)
- Fasting lipids: total cholesterol (TOT-C), 165 mg/dl; low-density lipoprotein cholesterol (LDL-C), 93 mg/dl; high-density lipoprotein cholesterol (HDL-C), 45 mg/dl; triglycerides (TG), 137 mg/dl
- Liver function tests: GOT, 19 U/L; GPT, 22 U/L; gamma-GT 28 mg/dL
- CPK = 134 U/L

Current Treatment

- Therapeutic lifestyle
- Enalapril/lercanidipine 20/20 mg 1 tablet h. 8.00
- Metformin/sitagliptin 850/50 mg 1 tablet h. 8.00 and 1 tablet h. 20.00
- ASA 100 mg 1 tablet after lunch
- Atorvastatin 20 mg 1 tablet h. 22.00
- Ezetimibe 10 mg 1 tablet h. 22.00

Treatment Evaluation

- No drug has been modified.
- No drug dose has changed.

Prescriptions

- Maintenance of therapeutic lifestyle measures
- Full haematochemistry and urinalysis

2.4 Follow-Up (Visit 3) at 1 Year

The patient reports a good adherence to the prescribed therapy and to the therapeutic lifestyle changes. She lost more weight. The glucose, lipid, and liver parameters strongly improved until normalization with further improvement in home BP values without subjective side effects.

Physical Examination

- Weight: 71.2 kg
- Height: 1.69 cm
- Body mass index (BMI): 24.9 kg/m^2
- Waist circumference: 91 cm
- Abdomen: normal, liver inferior border no more palpable below the costal margin

Haematological Profile

- Haemoglobin: 14.1 g/dL
- Haematocrit: 45 %
- Fasting plasma glucose: 121 mg/dL
- Glycated Haemoglobin (HbA1c): 52 mmol/mol (6.9 %)
- Fasting lipids: total cholesterol (TOT-C), 159 mg/dl; low-density lipoprotein cholesterol (LDL-C), 80 mg/dl; high-density lipoprotein cholesterol (HDL-C), 49 mg/dl; triglycerides (TG), 147 mg/dl
- Liver function tests: GOT 20 U/L, GPT 24 U/L, gamma-GT 31 mg/dL
- CPK = 153 U/L
- Electrolytes: sodium, 141 mEq/L; potassium, 3.8 mEq/L
- Serum uric acid: 5.1 mg/dL
- Renal function: urea, 21 mg/dl; creatinine, 0.7 mg/dL; creatinine clearance (Cockroft-Gault), 79.6 ml/min; estimated glomerular filtration rate (eGFR) (MDRD), 84 mL/min/1.73 m^2
- Urine analysis (dipstick): gravity 1026, pH 6.4, no glucose nor sediments
- Albuminuria: not detectable

Blood Pressure Profile

- Home BP (average): 110/76 mmHg
- Sitting BP: 126/78 mmHg (right arm); 125/76 mmHg (left arm)
- Standing BP: 124/75 mmHg at 1 min
- 24 h BP: 112/73 mmHg; HR, 72 bpm
- Daytime BP: 117/79 mmHg; HR, 76 bpm
- Night-time BP: 97/60 mmHg; HR, 62 bpm

Twenty-four-hour ambulatory blood pressure profile is illustrated in Fig. 2.4.

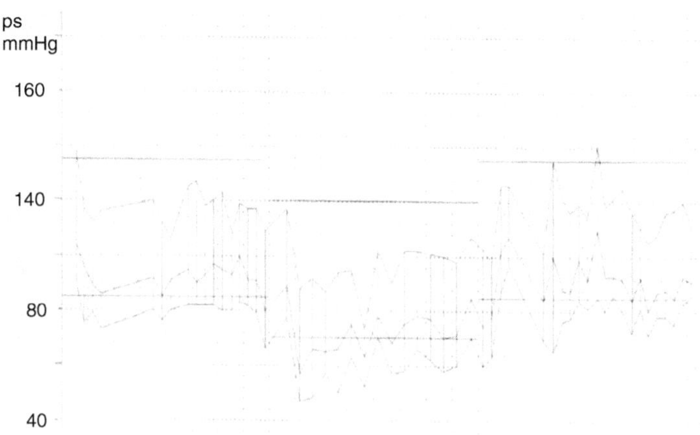

FIGURE 2.4 Patient post-treatment 24-h ambulatory blood pressure chart

Diagnostic Tests for Organ Damage or Associated Clinical Conditions

The patient has moderate to severe carotid atheroma. However, currently her blood pressure and her diabetes are perfectly controlled.

Current Treatment

- Therapeutic lifestyle
- Enalapril/lercanidipine 20/20 mg 1 tablet h. 8.00
- Metformin/sitagliptin 850/50 mg 1 tablet h. 8.00 and 1 tablet h. 20.00
- ASA 100 mg 1 tablet after lunch
- Atorvastatin 20 mg 1 tablet h. 22.00
- Ezetimibe 10 mg 1 tablet h. 22.00

Treatment Evaluation

- Therapeutic lifestyle (confirmed)
- Enalapril/lercanidipine 20/20 mg 1 tablet h. 8.00 (confirmed)

- Metformin/sitagliptin 850/50 mg 1 tablet h. 8.00 and 1 tablet h. 20.00 (confirmed)
- ASA 100 mg 1 tablet after lunch (confirmed)
- Atorvastatin 20 mg 1 tablet h. 22.00 (confirmed)
- Ezetimibe 10 mg 1 tablet h. 22.00 (confirmed)

Prescriptions

- Periodical BP evaluation at home according to recommendations from current guidelines
- Standard 12-ECG once a year
- Carotid ultrasound once a year

Which will be the most useful diagnostic test to repeat during the follow-up in this patient?

Possible answers are:

1. Electrocardiogram
2. Echocardiogram
3. Vascular Doppler ultrasound
4. Evaluation of renal parameters (e.g. creatininaemia, eGFR, ClCr, UACR)
5. Twenty-four-hour ambulatory BP monitoring

2.5 Discussion

Hypertension is one of the main determinants of cardiovascular risk in type 2 diabetes, and its management must be obtained with drugs not affecting lipid or glucose metabolism and preferably with a protecting effect of the kidney [1]. In the United Kingdom Prospective Diabetes Study (UKPDS), tight blood pressure control (average blood pressure 144/82 mmHg) reduced the risk of mortality by 32 % in patients with newly diagnosed type 2 diabetes compared to usual care (average blood pressure 154/87 mmHg) [2]. A recent meta-analysis of 40 randomized clinical trials enrolling 100.354 diabetic subjects concluded that each 10 mmHg reduction in systolic blood pressure is associated with a significantly lower risk of mortality (relative risk [RR], 0.87; 95 % CI, 0.78–0.96); absolute risk reduction (ARR) in events per 1000 patient-years (3.16; 95 % CI, 0.90–5.22), cardiovascular events (RR, 0.89 [95 % CI, 0.83–0.95]; ARR, 3.90 [95 % CI, 1.57–6.06]), coronary heart disease (RR, 0.88 [95 % CI, 0.80–0.98]; ARR, 1.81 [95 % CI, 0.35–3.11]), stroke (RR, 0.73 [95 % CI, 0.64–0.83]; ARR, 4.06 [95 % CI, 2.53–5.40]), albuminuria (RR, 0.83 [95 % CI, 0.79–0.87]; ARR, 9.33 [95 % CI, 7.13–11.37]), and retinopathy (RR, 0.87 [95 % CI, 0.76–0.99]; ARR, 2.23 [95 % CI, 0.15–4.04]) [3].

In the clinical case reported above, the patient had an uncontrolled blood pressure, especially early in the night and in the morning. Moreover, she suffered from sudden weakness, most likely related to hypoglycaemia rather than low blood pressure, because the 24-h ABPM did not show any hypotension episode. Consequently, we respected the priority of BP improvement, but we had also to improve the type 2 diabetes management. Therefore, since our patient was treated with glibenclamide, a sulphonylurea potentially associated with hypoglycaemic episodes and weight gain, we substituted it with sitagliptin, a dipeptidyl peptidase (DPP)-4 inhibitor, usually not associated with these side effects [4]. In particular, sitagliptin cardiovascular safety has been clearly demonstrated in the large Trial Evaluating Cardiovascular Outcomes with Sitagliptin (TECOS) trial, enrolling *14,735* type 2 diabetic subjects [5] (Fig. 2.5).

Finally, we also optimize the patient LDL level increasing the efficacy of the lipid-lowering drugs prescribed, in line with that suggested by the latest ESC/EAS guidelines [6].

The antihypertensive approach with enalapril and lercanidipine in one pill is based on the purpose to use metabolically neutral (or mildly improving) drugs, both associated to nephroprotection, and acting on the 24 h [7]. The global approach on more risk factors in type 2 diabetes seems in fact to be the most effective in terms of reduction of cardiovascular diseases and all-cause death risk, as clearly shown by the STENO-2 trial [8].

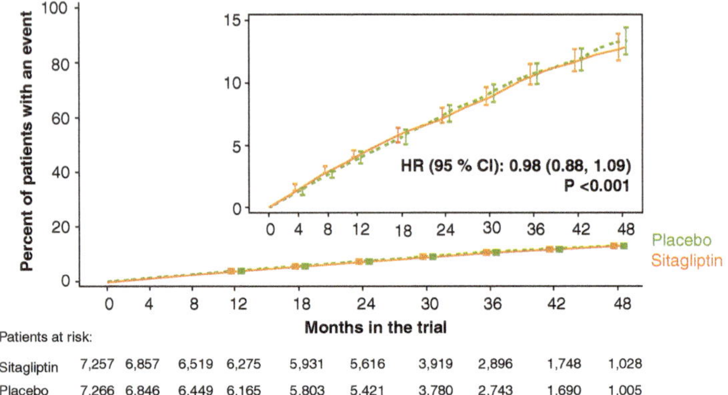

FIGURE 2.5 Primary composite cardiovascular outcome (cardiovascular death, nonfatal MI, nonfatal stroke, hospitalization for unstable angina) in the TECOS

Take-Home Messages

- Type 2 diabetes is highly prevalent in general population and among hypertensive subjects.
- Hypertension is one of the main determinants of cardiovascular disease risk in type 2 diabetes.
- When treating type 2 diabetes patients, it is relevant to choose antihypertensive drugs without metabolic interference with glucose and lipid metabolism but also with nephroprotective effects.
- Blockers of the renin-angiotensin-aldosterone system and calcium antagonists are usually preferred for the management of hypertensive patients with metabolic syndrome.
- The global management of type 2 diabetes, with parallel improvement of LDL cholesterolaemia, blood pressure, and glucose metabolism, is the one associated with the better outcomes in terms of cardiovascular disease prevention.

References

1. Mancia G, Fagard R, Narkiewicz K, Redon J, Zanchetti A, Bohm M, et al. 2013 ESH/ESC Guidelines for the management of arterial hypertension: the Task Force for the management of arterial

hypertension of the European Society of Hypertension (ESH) and of the European Society of Cardiology (ESC). J Hypertens. 2013;31(7):1281–357.

2. UK Prospective Diabetes Study Group. Tight blood pressure control and risk of macrovascular and microvascular complications in type 2 diabetes: UKPDS 38. BMJ. 1998; 317:703–13.
3. Emdin CA, Rahimi K, Neal B, Callender T, Perkovic V, Patel A. Blood pressure lowering in type 2 diabetes: a systematic review and meta-analysis. JAMA. 2015;313(6):603–15.
4. Deacon CF, Lebovitz HE. Comparative review of dipeptidyl peptidase-4 inhibitors and sulphonylureas. Diabetes Obes Metab. 2016;18(4):333–47.
5. Green JB, Bethel MA, Armstrong PW, Buse JB, Engel SS, Garg J, Josse R, Kaufman KD, Koglin J, Korn S, Lachin JM, McGuire DK, Pencina MJ, Standl E, Stein PP, Suryawanshi S, Van de Werf F, Peterson ED, Holman RR, TECOS Study Group. Effect of Sitagliptin on Cardiovascular Outcomes in Type 2 Diabetes. N Engl J Med. 2015;373(3):232–42.
6. European Association for Cardiovascular Prevention & Rehabilitation, Reiner Z, Catapano AL, De Backer G, Graham I, Taskinen MR, Wiklund O, Agewall S, Alegria E, Chapman MJ, Durrington P, Erdine S, Halcox J, Hobbs R, Kjekshus J, Filardi PP, Riccardi G, Storey RF, Wood D, ESC Committee for Practice Guidelines (CPG) 2008–2010 and 2010–2012 Committees. ESC/EAS Guidelines for the management of dyslipidaemias: the Task Force for the management of dyslipidaemias of the European Society of Cardiology (ESC) and the European Atherosclerosis Society (EAS). Eur Heart J. 2011;32(14):1769–818.
7. Borghi C, Cicero AF. Rationale for the use of a fixed-dose combination in the management of hypertension: efficacy and tolerability of lercanidipine/enalapril. Clin Drug Investig. 2010;30(12):843–54.
8. Gaede P, Lund-Andersen H, Parving HH, Pedersen O. Effect of a multifactorial intervention on mortality in type 2 diabetes. N Engl J Med. 2008;358(6):580–91.

Chapter 3
Clinical Case 3: Patient with Essential Hypertension and Familial Hypercholesterolaemia

3.1 Clinical Case Presentation

Man, 48 years old, entrepreneur, non-smoker, and overall healthy. One year ago, after the third intercontinental flight in a month, he experienced a syncope and was recovered in an emergency department. During the short permanence in the emergency room, a standard 12-lead ECG and a brain TC did not show any pathological signs. The patient refused to continue the test because he felt fine, but the BP at the admission was 182/96 mmHg and at the discharge 168/92 mmHg. Then he refused to take any kind of medicine and to be further visited.

He comes to our centre 1 year after because a persistent headache associated with a feeling of dizziness slows his affairs.

Family History

The patient relatives were not hypertensive nor diabetics; however his mother and his brother were hypercholesterolaemic. The mother, non-smoker and overweight but not diabetic, had the first myocardial infarction at the age of 54 and then died because of a second myocardial infarction at the age of 61. The brother, smoker, died because of a stroke at 63 years, though he had taken lipid-lowering drugs from the age of 50.

A.F.G. Cicero, *Hypertension and Metabolic Cardiovascular Risk Factors*, Practical Case Studies in Hypertension Management, DOI 10.1007/978-3-319-39504-3_3,

Clinical History

The patient claims to be "healthy" and to feel fit. The only episode of interest he tells is about a syncope he had 1 year ago, associated with high blood pressure, which he attributed to psychophysical stress. His family history is impressive. He is not a snorer (information confirmed by the wife) and he has no nocturia. He usually did not measure BP at home. The 12-lead standard ECG done in the morning of the visit was overall normal. The last haematochemistry shows a severe hypercholesterolaemia, associated with a normal renal function.

Physical Examination

- Weight: 76.4 kg.
- Height: 1.82 cm.
- Body mass index (BMI): 23.1 kg/m^2.
- Waist circumference: 93 cm.
- Respiration: auscultation of the chest reveals clear lung fields and no murmurs or rubs.
- Heart sounds: regular rhythm, no accessory murmurs.
- Resting pulse: regular, 69 bpm.
- Carotid arteries: no bruit on auscultation.
- Femoral and foot arteries: all pulses present and normosphygmic.
- Abdomen: overall normal, no pain at superficial and deep palpation.
- Hand: evident tendon xanthomas (Fig. 3.1).

Haematological Profile

- Haemoglobin: 14.7 g/dL
- Haematocrit: 44 %
- Fasting plasma glucose: 97 mg/dL

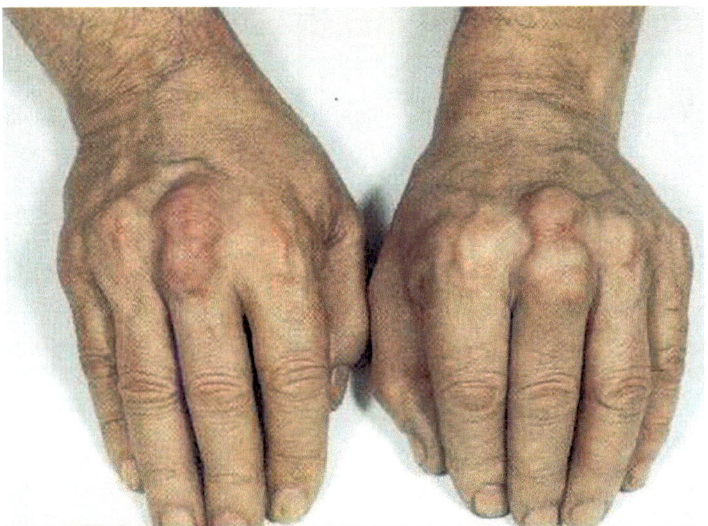

FIGURE 3.1 Patient tendon xanthomas

- Fasting lipids: total cholesterol (TOT-C), 301 mg/dl; low-density lipoprotein cholesterol (LDL-C), 226 mg/dl; high-density lipoprotein cholesterol (HDL-C), 45 mg/dl; triglycerides (TG), 149 mg/dl
- Electrolytes: sodium, 140 mEq/L; potassium, 3.9 mEq/L
- Serum uric acid: 5.2 mg/dL
- Renal function: urea, 21 mg/dl; creatinine, 0.9 mg/dL; creatinine clearance (Cockroft-Gault), 107.9 ml/min; estimated glomerular filtration rate (eGFR) (MDRD), 96 mL/min/1.73 m^2
- Urine analysis (dipstick): gravity 1022, pH 6.7, no glucose nor sediments
- Albuminuria: 21 mg/24 h
- Liver function tests: GOT, 24 U/L; GPT, 27 U/L; gamma-GT, 27 mg/dL
- Thyroid function tests: in the normal range

Blood Pressure Profile

- Home BP (average): usually not measured
- Sitting BP: 162/96 mmHg (right arm); 160/94 mmHg (left arm)
- Standing BP: 160/94 mmHg at 1 min
- 24 h BP: not known
- Daytime BP: not known
- Night-time BP: not known

Twelve-Lead Electrocardiogram

The standard 12-lead ECG executed the day of the visit shows sinus rhythm, PR < 0.2 s, QRS < 0.1 s, normal progression of R wave, ST isoelectric, and T waves positive in all precordial derivations. Therefore, it is overall normal (Fig. 3.2).

Current Treatment

- None.

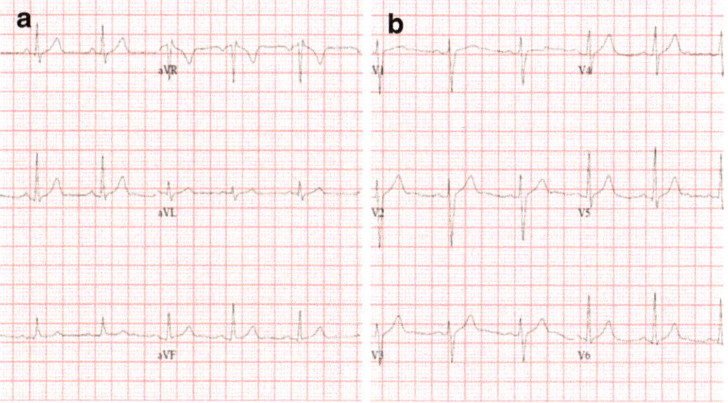

FIGURE 3.2 Patient baseline standard 12-lead ECG

Diagnosis

Grade II hypertension in heterozygous familial hypercholesterolaemia (as per Dutch Lipid Score >8, Table 3.1), apparently not complicated by left ventricular hypertrophy and microalbuminuria.

In the light of the available information, what is the estimated cardiovascular risk of the patient?

Possible answers are:

1. Low
2. Medium
3. High
4. Very high

Global Cardiovascular Risk Stratification

The patient has two additive risk factors (hypercholesterolaemia and family history of early cardiovascular events); therefore, the ESH/ESC guidelines would be used to evaluate the patient as at moderate to high risk [1]. Though the condition of familial hypercholesterolaemia is however associated with a maximally increased cardiovascular risk, the parallel presence of hypertension made even more serious the situation [2].

Which is the best therapeutic option for this patient at this step?

Possible answers are:

1. Start immediately with an antihypertensive drug without negative effects on lipid metabolism (e.g. dihydropyridinic calcium antagonist or RAS blocker).

TABLE 3.1 The Dutch Lipid Score of our patient is 10

	Criteria	Score
Family history	First-degree relative known with premature CAD* and/or first-degree relative with LDL-C >95th centile	1
	First-degree relative with Tx and/or children <18 with LDL-C >95th centile	2
Clinical history	Patient has premature CAD*	2
	Patient has premature cerebral/ peripheral vascular disease	1
Physical examination	Tx	6
	Arcus cornealis below the age of 45 years	4
LDL-C	>8.5 mmol/L (more than ~330 mg/dL)	8
	6.5–8.4 mmol/L (~250–329 mg/dL)	5
	5.0–6.4 mmol/L (~190–249 mg/dL)	3
	4.0–4.9 mmol/L (~155–189 mg/dL)	1
Definite FH		Score >8
Probable FH		Score 6-8
Possible FH		Score 3-5
No diagnosis		Score <3

*Definite Myocardial Infarction or sudden death in Father or first-degree male relative under age 55 or Mother or first-degree female relative under age 65

2. Start immediately with an antihypertensive drug without negative effects on lipid metabolism (e.g. dihydropyridinic calcium antagonist or RAS blocker) and a lipid-lowering treatment (e.g. statin).
3. Start with a beta-blocker.
4. Start with a full-dosed thiazide.
5. Start with a lipid-lowering treatment (e.g. statin) only.

Treatment Evaluation

- Amlodipine 5 mg in 1 tablet h. 8.00
- Atorvastatin 20 mg 1 tablet h. 22.00

Prescriptions

- Therapeutic lifestyle prescription, in particular the patient was instructed to follow the general indications of a Mediterranean diet, avoiding excessive intake of dairy products and red meat, increasing the intake of vegetables, and reducing as possible the consumption of salt. Moreover, he was also encouraged to increase his physical activity by walking briskly for 20 to 30 min, three to five times per week, or by cycling.
- Haematochemistry to evaluate the statin efficacy and safety (to be done after 8–10 weeks of treatment, if well tolerated).
- 24 h ambulatory blood pressure.
- Carotid echo-colour Doppler examination.

3.2 Follow-Up (Visit 1) at 6 Weeks

The patient affirms to have regularly taken the prescribed pills that are well tolerated. He also states to have put stronger attention to his diet, significantly reducing the content of salt, and sensibly improved the weekly physical activity, walking at least 45 min each day.

Physical Examination

- Overall unchanged, when compared with the previous visit.

Blood Pressure Profile

- Home BP (average): 143/76 mmHg
- Sitting BP: 149/80 mmHg
- Standing BP: 148/78 mmHg
- 24 h BP: 137/83 mmHg
- Daytime BP: 148/88 mmHg
- Night-time BP: 112/70 mmHg

Twenty-four-hour ambulatory blood pressure profile (with amlodipine 5 mg/day) is illustrated in Fig. 3.3. 71 % of diurnal

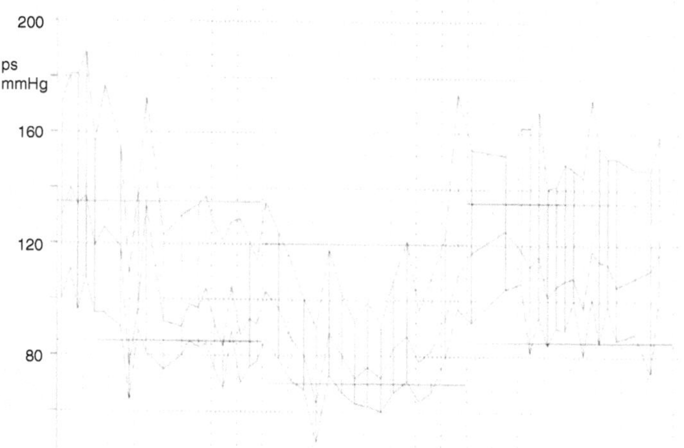

FIGURE 3.3 24-h ambulatory blood pressure profile during amlodipine 5 mg/day treatment

SBP measurements, and 55 of the DBP ones are above normal.

Current Treatment

- Therapeutic lifestyle
- Amlodipine 5 mg in 1 tablet h. 8.00
- Atorvastatin 20 mg 1 tablet h. 22.00

Diagnostic Tests for Organ Damage or Associated Clinical Conditions

The carotid ultrasound examination shows diffuse intima-media thickening with IMT = 1.2–1.3 mm in different districts, with a calcified carotid plaque in the right common carotid artery (Fig. 3.4).

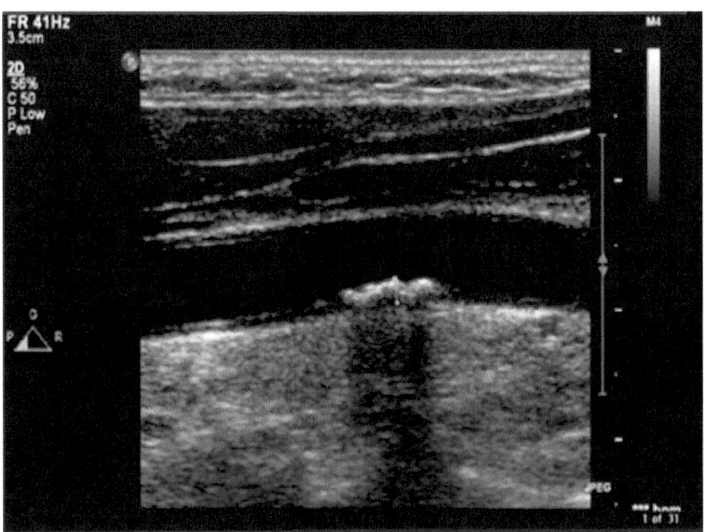

FIGURE 3.4 Patient's right carotid artery ultrasound

Diagnosis

Grade II hypertension in heterozygous familial hypercholesterolaemia, complicated by carotid atheroma.

In the light of the available information, what is the estimated cardiovascular risk of the patient?

Possible answers are:

1. Low
2. Medium
3. High
4. Very high

Global Cardiovascular Risk Stratification

BP has improved but is yet not adequately controlled, and the estimated risk for the patient is high, in particular because of the presence of target organ damage (carotid atherosclerosis) [1]. The discovery of carotid atherosclerosis modifies the LDL-C target for this patient to a level that is not achievable with atorvastatin alone [3].

Which is the best therapeutic option for this patient at this step?

Possible answers are:

1. Add a RAS blocker.
2. Add a RAS blocker and another lipid-lowering treatment (e.g. ezetimibe).
3. Start with a beta-blocker.
4. Start with a full-dosed thiazide.
5. Add a RAS blocker and double the atorvastatin dose.

Treatment Evaluation

- Therapeutic lifestyle
- Perindopril 5 mg/amlodipine 5 mg in 1 tablet h. 8.00
- Atorvastatin 20 mg 1 tablet h. 22.00
- Ezetimibe 10 mg 1 tablet h. 22.00

Prescriptions

- Intensification of therapeutic lifestyle measures, with particular attention to physical activity
- Lipid pattern with liver transaminases, gamma-GT, and CPK (to be performed after 8–12 weeks)

3.3 Follow-Up (Visit 2) at 3 Months

The patient reports further improvement in home BP values without subjective side effects. He continues to care about his diet, and he began to practise some physical activity (even if not so intensively as prescribed).

Physical Examination

- No changes compared to the previous visits.

Blood Pressure Profile

- Home BP (average): 135/74 mmHg
- Sitting BP: 138/82 mmHg
- Standing BP: 136/82 mmHg

Current Treatment

- Perindopril 5 mg/amlodipine 5 mg in 1 tablet h. 8.00
- Atorvastatin 20 mg 1 tablet h. 22.00
- Ezetimibe 10 mg 1 tablet h. 22.00

Treatment Evaluation

- No drug has been modified.
- No drug dose has been changed.

Prescriptions

- Maintenance of therapeutic lifestyle measures
- ABPM
- Full haematochemistry and urinalysis

3.4 Follow-Up (Visit 3) at 1 Year

The patient reports a good adherence to the prescribed therapy and to the therapeutic lifestyle changes. He lost some weight. The glucose, lipid, and liver parameters strongly improved until normalization with further improvement in home BP values without subjective side effects.

Physical Examination

- Weight: 74.8 kg
- Height: 1.82 cm
- Body mass index (BMI): 22.6 kg/m^2
- Waist circumference: 91 cm
- No changes in thoracic and abdominal examination

Haematological Profile

- Fasting plasma glucose: 91 mg/dL
- Fasting lipids: total cholesterol (TOT-C), 162 mg/dl; low-density lipoprotein cholesterol (LDL-C), 89 mg/dl; high-density lipoprotein cholesterol (HDL-C), 47 mg/dl; triglycerides (TG), 132 mg/dl

- Liver function tests: GOT 24 U/L, GPT 29 U/L, gamma-GT 31 mg/dL
- CPK = 181 U/L
- Albuminuria: 11 mg/24 h

Blood Pressure Profile

- Home BP (average): 120/74 mmHg
- Sitting BP: 136/78 mmHg (right arm); 135/76 mmHg (left arm)
- Standing BP: 134/77 mmHg at 1 min
- 24 h BP: 121/67 mmHg; HR: 68 bpm
- Daytime BP: 128/80 mmHg; HR, 72 bpm
- Night-time BP: 111/66 mmHg; HR, 60 bpm

Twenty-four-hour ambulatory blood pressure profile is illustrated in Fig. 3.5.

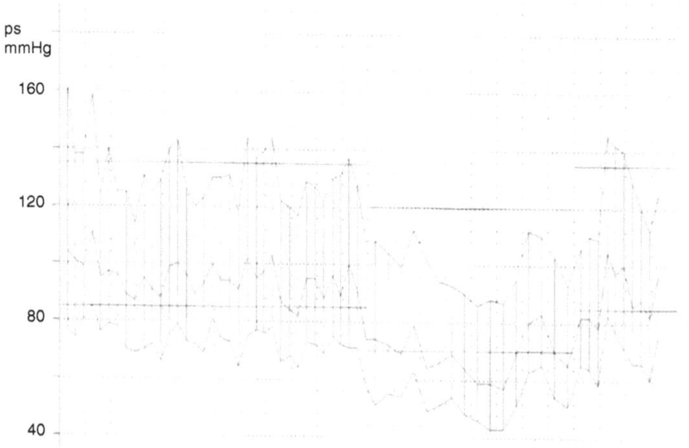

FIGURE 3.5 24-h ambulatory blood pressure profile after treatment intensification

Diagnostic Tests for Organ Damage or Associated Clinical Conditions

Albuminuria that was already in the normal range decreases to a lower value; however the risk of the patient remains high because of the permanence of other signs of target organ damage (carotid plaques).

Current Treatment

- Therapeutic lifestyle
- Perindopril 5 mg/amlodipine 5 mg in 1 tablet h. 8.00
- Atorvastatin 20 mg 1 tablet h. 22.00
- Ezetimibe 10 mg 1 tablet h. 22.00

Treatment Evaluation

- Therapeutic lifestyle (confirmed)
- Perindopril 5 mg/amlodipine 5 mg in 1 tablet h. 8.00 (confirmed)
- Atorvastatin 20 mg 1 tablet h. 22.00 (confirmed)
- Ezetimibe 10 mg 1 tablet h. 22.00 (confirmed)

Prescriptions

- Periodical BP evaluation at home according to recommendations from current guidelines
- Standard 12-ECG once a year
- Carotid ultrasound once a year

Which will be the most useful diagnostic test to repeat during the follow-up in this patient?

Possible answers are:

1. Electrocardiogram
2. Echocardiogram

3. Vascular Doppler ultrasound
4. Evaluation of renal parameters (e.g. creatininaemia, eGFR, ClCr, UACR)
5. Twenty-four-hour ambulatory BP monitoring

3.5 Discussion

Familial hypercholesterolaemia is a relatively common severe disease of the lipid metabolism that per se dramatically increases the risk of coronary and cerebrovascular events. Currently, with the help of the Dutch Lipid Score, it is very easy to detect these patients.

The relationship between hypercholesterolaemia and hypertension is strong. They are often present in the same patient, but hypercholesterolaemia could precede the appearance of hypertension [4]. In particular, the level of LDL-C (usually very high in subjects affected by familial hypercholesterolaemia) is directly related to the expression of the AT1 receptors (Fig. 3.6).

The clinical case here described is prototypical. Despite a relevant family history of early cardiovascular events, the patient did not care about his health until the appearance of some symptoms. On the other side, with the Dutch Lipid Score, each physician could have been able to recognize his metabolic disorders, especially because of the evidence of tendinous xanthomas that are nearly pathognomonic of familial hypercholesterolaemia.

As it regards the choice of the antihypertensive treatment, in this kind of patients, the guidelines suggest to prefer metabolically neutral drugs, like renin-angiotensin-aldosterone system blocking drug and/or calcium antagonists, maintaining thiazides or beta-blockers as second choices, when not strictly required [1].

A combined treatment has been chosen in order to improve the ability (and the will) of the patient to regularly

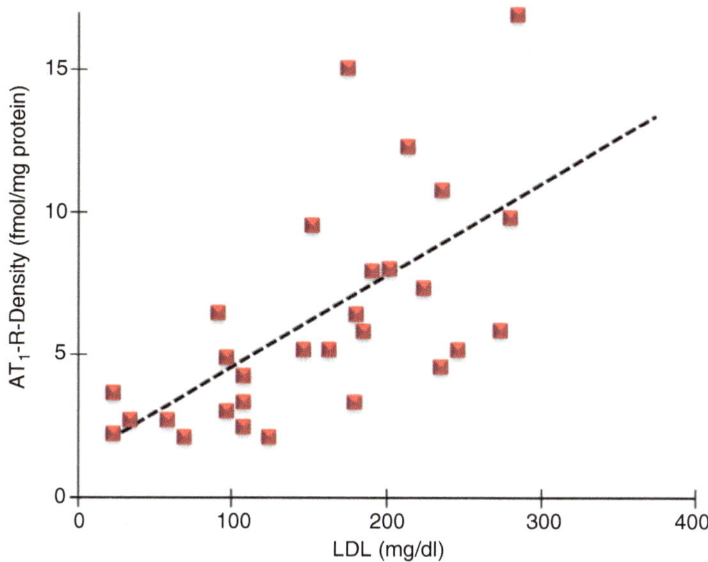

FIGURE 3.6 Regression analysis of plasma LDL concentration and platelet AT1 receptor density in men (Modified from Nickenig et al. [5])

take his daily therapy. The association of amlodipine and atorvastatin was chosen as the first step of therapy, since the Anglo-Scandinavian Cardiac Outcomes Trial-Lipid Lowering Arm (ASCOT-LLA) study clearly showed that this approach was highly effective in reducing cardiovascular disease risk in hypertensive hypercholesterolaemic subjects [6]. The addition of perindopril to the antihypertensive treatment improved the patient BP to optimal level.

Doubling the statin dose in this case would have been not useful to reach the LDL-C target suggested by the last EAS/ ESC guidelines [3], so we preferred to add in therapy ezetimibe, whose effect is synergistic with the one of statins, and, one more time, the choice was successful.

Take-Home Messages

- Familial hypercholesterolaemia is a severe disease of the lipid metabolism that per se dramatically increases the risk of coronary and cerebrovascular events.
- The overlapping of familial hypercholesterolemia with hypertension strongly increases the risk to develop hypertension-related complications (in particular cardiovascular events).
- The exposition to hypercholesterolaemia since young age could be a risk factor for the development of hypertension.
- When treating familial hypercholesterolemia patients, it is relevant to choose antihypertensive drugs without metabolic interference with lipid metabolism.
- The result of the ASCOT-LLT suggests that the association of atorvastatin with perindopril and amlodipine is an efficacious way to significantly reduce the cardiovascular disease risk of hypercholesterolaemic hypertensive patients.

References

1. Mancia G, Fagard R, Narkiewicz K, Redon J, Zanchetti A, Bohm M, et al. 2013 ESH/ESC Guidelines for the management of arterial hypertension: the Task Force for the management of arterial hypertension of the European Society of Hypertension (ESH) and of the European Society of Cardiology (ESC). J Hypertens. 2013;31(7):1281–357.
2. Wong B, Villa G, Kutikova L, Kruse G, Ray KK, Mata P, Bruckert E. The Magnitude of Increased Cardiovascular (Cv) Risk Associated with Familial Hypercholesterolemia (Fh) for use in Economic Analyses. Value Health. 2015;18(7):A340.
3. European Association for Cardiovascular Prevention & Rehabilitation, Reiner Z, Catapano AL, De Backer G, Graham I,

Taskinen MR, Wiklund O, Agewall S, Alegria E, Chapman MJ, Durrington P, Erdine S, Halcox J, Hobbs R, Kjekshus J, Filardi PP, Riccardi G, Storey RF, Wood D, ESC Committee for Practice Guidelines (CPG) 2008–2010 and 2010–2012 Committees. ESC/EAS Guidelines for the management of dyslipidaemias: the Task Force for the management of dyslipidaemias of the European Society of Cardiology (ESC) and the European Atherosclerosis Society (EAS). Eur Heart J. 2011;32(14):1769–818.

4. Borghi C, Cicero AF, Saragoni S, Buda S, Cristofori C, Lilli P, Degli Esposti L. Rate of control of LDL cholesterol and incident hypertension requiring antihypertensive treatment in hypercholesterolemic subjects in daily clinical practice. Ann Med. 2014;46(2):97–102.
5. Nickenig G, Baumer AT, Temur Y, Kebben D, Jockenhovel F, Bohm M. Statin-sensitive dysregulated AT1 receptor function and density in hypercholesterolemic mend. Circulation. 1999;100:2131–4.
6. Sever P, Dahlöf B, Poulter N, Wedel H, Beevers G, Caulfield M, Collins R, Kjeldsen S, Kristinsson A, McInnes G, Mehlsen J, Nieminem M, O'Brien E. Ostergren J; ASCOT Steering Committee Members. Potential synergy between lipid-lowering and blood-pressure-lowering in the Anglo-Scandinavian Cardiac Outcomes Trial. Eur Heart J. 2006;27(24):2982–8.

Chapter 4
Clinical Case 4: Patient with Essential Hypertension and Hypertriglyceridaemia

4.1 Clinical Case Presentation

Man, 59 years old, never a smoker, and mildly overweight from the young age, with nearly no physical activity (his working life is sedentary as the leisure one). He knows he is hypertensive since 20 years when his GPs began to treat him with atenolol 100 mg 1 cp in the morning. He remembers that his GPs gave him this drug because he also had a mild tachycardia. During the last winter, his blood pressure further increased and his old GPs added in therapy hydrochlorothiazide 25 mg in the morning. His blood pressure is relatively well controlled with this therapy, but he comes to our observation after the suggestion of his new GP, worried about potential side effects of beta-blockers and diuretics on his erectile function.

Family History

The patient's family is not particularly characteristic. No one in the family died nor was affected by early cardiovascular diseases. No one was diabetic. His father was mildly overweight, while his mother is hypertriglyceridaemic (95 years old, overall in good shape) as well as his younger sister (54 years old).

A.F.G. Cicero, *Hypertension and Metabolic Cardiovascular Risk Factors*, Practical Case Studies in Hypertension Management, DOI 10.1007/978-3-319-39504-3_4,

Clinical History

The patient is in primary prevention for cardiovascular disease and is not diabetic. He has an overall healthy diet, even if too rich when compared with his physical activity. No test was specifically carried out until now to evaluate eventual target organ damages. His wife says that he sometimes snores, but apparently without episodes of apnoea. On the other side, he says that his sexual performance have significantly impaired from the winter. He tried to suspend atenolol, but he felt a reappraisal of the previously experienced tachycardia. He also knows he is hypertriglyceridaemic, but he does not care about it because he knows that it is a "family trait" and his hypertriglyceridaemic mother is a healthy elderly woman.

Physical Examination

- Weight: 81.4 kg.
- Height: 1.75 cm.
- Body mass index (BMI): 26.6 kg/m^2.
- Waist circumference: 99 cm.
- Respiration: auscultation of the chest reveals clear lung fields and no murmurs or rubs.
- Heart sounds: regular rhythm, no accessory murmurs.
- Resting pulse: regular, 70 bpm.
- Carotid arteries: no bruit on auscultation.
- Femoral and foot arteries: all pulses present and normosphygmic.
- Abdomen: globular, liver inferior border palpable 2.5 cm below the costal margin.

Haematological Profile

- Haemoglobin: 14.2 g/dL
- Haematocrit: 44 %
- Fasting plasma glucose: 99 mg/dL

- Fasting lipids: total cholesterol (TOT-C), 163 mg/dl; non-high-density lipoprotein cholesterol (non-HDL-C), 122 mg/dl; high-density lipoprotein cholesterol (HDL-C), 41 mg/dl; triglycerides (TG), 721 mg/dl
- Electrolytes: sodium, 140 mEq/L; potassium, 3.9 mEq/L
- Serum uric acid: 5.8 mg/dL
- Renal function: urea, 18 mg/dl; creatinine, 1.0 mg/dL; creatinine clearance (Cockroft-Gault), 91.1 ml/min; estimated glomerular filtration rate (eGFR) (MDRD), 76 mL/min/1.73 m^2
- Urine analysis (dipstick): gravity 1018, pH 6.9, no glucose nor sediments
- Albuminuria: <10 mg/24 h
- Liver function tests: GOT, 33 U/L; GPT, 39 U/L; gamma-GT, 51 mg/dL (suggestive of a nonalcoholic fatty liver disease)
- Thyroid function tests: in the normal range

Blood Pressure Profile

- Home BP (average): 130/80 mmHg
- Sitting BP: 134/84 mmHg (right arm); 135/86 mmHg (left arm)
- Standing BP: 132/80 mmHg at 1 min
- Twenty-four-hour BP: 132/84 mmHg; HR, 71 bpm
- Daytime BP: 132/83 mmHg; HR, 73 bpm
- Night-time BP: 132/85 mmHg; HR, 68 bpm

Twenty-four-hour ambulatory blood pressure profile is illustrated in Fig. 4.1.

Twelve-Lead Electrocardiogram

The standard 12-lead ECG shows signs of left ventricular hypertrophy as per Sokolow index value (Fig. 4.2).

Current Treatment

- Atenolol 100 mg 1 tablet h. 8.00
- Hydrochlorothiazide 25 mg 1 tablet h. 8.00

Diagnosis

Grade I hypertension and familial hypertriglyceridaemia, complicated by electrocardiographically diagnosed left ventricular hypertrophy

In the light of the available information, what is the estimated cardiovascular risk of the patient?

Possible answers are:

1. Low
2. Medium
3. High
4. Very high

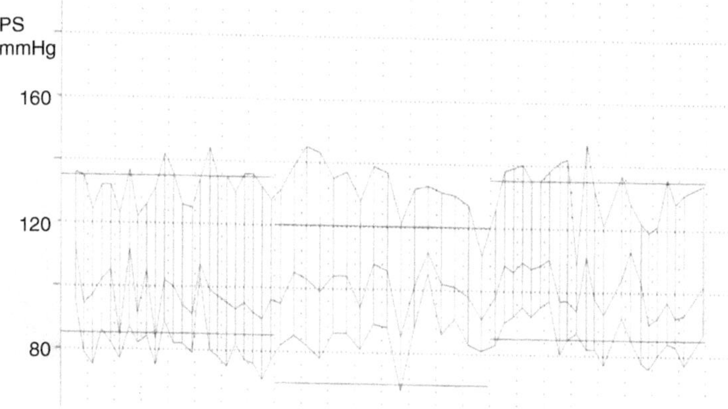

FIGURE 4.1 Baseline patient 24-h ambulatory blood pressure chart

Global Cardiovascular Risk Stratification

The patient has more than two additional risk factors, but also left ventricular hypertrophy, so that he has to be classified as a subject with high added cardiovascular risk [1].

Which is the best therapeutic option in this patient at this step?

Possible answers are:

1. Add another drug class (e.g. dihydropyridinic calcium antagonist).
2. Switch from atenolol to another beta-blocker with less impact on erectile function (e.g. nebivolol).
3. Switch from the beta-blocker to an ACE inhibitor.
4. Switch from the beta-blocker to an ARB.
5. Switch from the thiazide diuretic to an ACE inhibitor.

Treatment Evaluation

- Nebivolol 5 mg 1 tablet h. 8.00
- Hydrochlorothiazide 25 mg 1 tablet h. 8.00

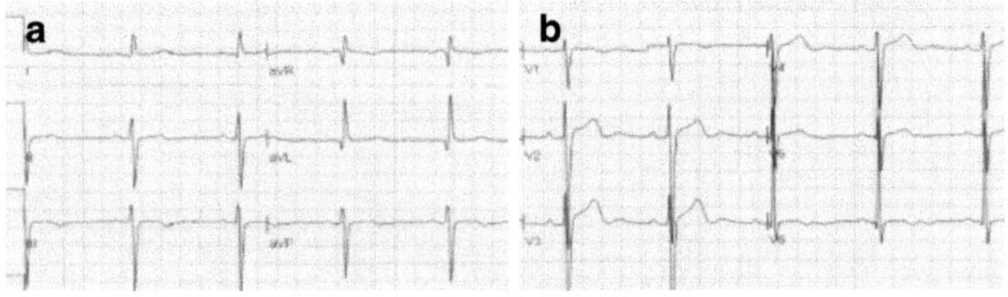

FIGURE 4.2 (**a**, **b**) – Patient baseline standard 12-lead ECG. Left ventricular hypertrophy with Sokolow index = 38 mm

Prescriptions

- Therapeutic lifestyle prescription, in particular the patient was instructed to follow the general indications of a Mediterranean diet, avoiding excessive intake of dairy products and red meat, increasing the intake of vegetables, and reducing as possible the consumption of salt. Moreover, he was also encouraged to increase his physical activity by walking briskly for 20–30 min, three to five times per week, or by cycling.
- Liver ultrasound.

4.2 Follow-Up (Visit 1) at 6 Weeks

The patient is satisfied with the reduction of tablet number to be taken daily and claims that his BP at home is "perfectly controlled". He states that the prescribed diet is very similar to the one he already followed before, but he tried to improve his daily physical activity. He had the perception of a mild improvement of his erectile function, but he is not yet so sure.

Physical Examination

- Overall unchanged, when compared with the previous visit. The patient lost 0.4 kg.

Blood Pressure Profile

- Home BP (average): 130/80 mmHg
- Sitting BP: 132/82 mmHg
- Standing BP: 132/80 mmHg

Current Treatment

- Therapeutic lifestyle
- Nebivolol 5 mg 1 tablet h. 8.00
- Hydrochlorothiazide 25 mg 1 tablet h. 8.00

Diagnostic Tests for Organ Damage or Associated Clinical Conditions

The International Index of Erectile Function Questionnaire (IIEF-5) is the worldwide-validated specific questionnaire to investigate erectile dysfunction severity (Fig. 4.3) [2]. The patient IIEF-5 score is 13, corresponding to a mild-to-moderate erectile dysfunction.

The liver ultrasound with ultrasound elastography images shows grade 2 fatty liver with decrease in shearing velocity (0.80 m/s, where the shearing velocity in the normal liver parenchyma is 1 m/s) (Fig. 4.4).

Diagnosis

Grade I hypertension and familial hypertriglyceridaemia, complicated by electrocardiographically diagnosed left ventricular hypertrophy and nonalcoholic fatty liver disease (NAFLD).

In the light of the available information, what is the estimated cardiovascular risk of the patient?

Possible answers are:

1. Low
2. Medium
3. High
4. Very high

The IIEF-5 questionnnaire (SHIM)

Please encircle the response that best describes you for the following five questions:

Over the past 6 months:					
1.How do you rate your confidence that you could get and keep an erection?	Very low 1	Low 2	Moderate 3	High 4	Very high 5
2. When you had erections with sexual stimulation, how often were your erections hard enough for penetration?	Almost never or never 1	A few times (much less then half the time) 2	Sometimes (about half the time) 3	Most times (much more then half the time) 4	Almost always or always 5
3.During sexual intercourse,how often werw you able to maintain your erection after you had penetrated your partner?	Almost never or never 1	A few times (much less then half the time) 2	Sometimes (about half the time) 3	Most times (much more then half the time) 4	Almost always or always 5
4.During sexual intercourse,how difficult was it to maintain your erection to completion of intercourse?	Extremely difficult 1	Very difficult 2	Difficult 3	Slightly difficult 4	Not difficult 5
5.When you attempted sexual intercourse,how often was it satisfactory for you?	Almost never or never 1	A few times (much less then half the time) 2	Sometimes (about half the time) 3	Most times (much more then half the time) 4	Almost always or always 5

Total score: ____________

1–7:Sevese ED 8–11:Moderate ED 12–16: MIld-Moderete ED 17–21: Mild ED 22–25: No ED

FIGURE 4.3 Standard International Index of Erectile Function Questionnaire (IIEF-5)

Global Cardiovascular Risk Stratification

The patient has more than two additional risk factors, but also left ventricular hypertrophy, so that he has to be classified as a subject with high added cardiovascular risk [1]. However, the risk of the patient could be higher, because of

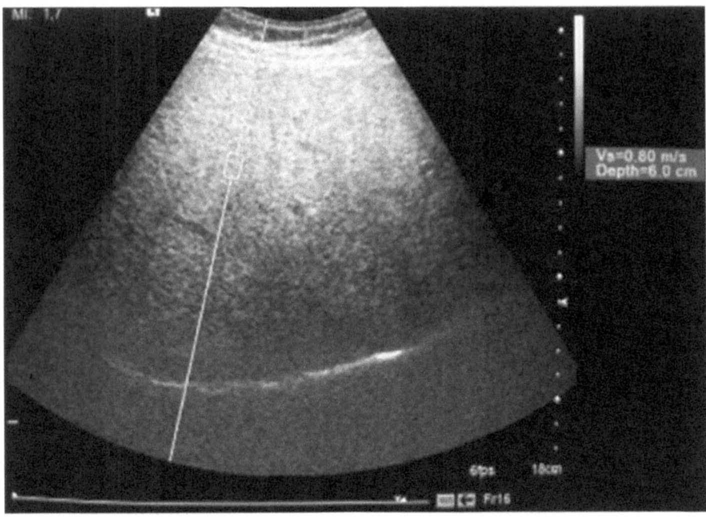

FIGURE 4.4 Patient liver ultrasound elastography image

the presence of erectile dysfunction and NALFD, not yet included among the consolidated risk factors by the last ESH-ESC guidelines [1].

Which is the best therapeutic option for this patient at this step?

Possible answers are:

1. Add another drug class (e.g. dihydropyridinic calcium antagonist).
2. Switch from the beta-blocker to an ARB.
3. Switch from the beta-blocker to an ACE inhibitor.
4. Switch from the thiazide diuretic to an ARB.
5. Switch from the thiazide diuretic to an ACE inhibitor.

Treatment Evaluation

- Therapeutic lifestyle
- Nebivolol 5 mg 1 tablet h. 8.00
- Telmisartan 40 mg 1 tablet h. 20.00 (in spite of hydrochlorothiazide)

Prescriptions

- Intensification of therapeutic lifestyle measures, with particular attention to physical activity
- Lipid pattern with liver transaminases; gamma-GT, and CPK

4.3 Follow-Up (Visit 2) at 3 Months

The patient reports an improvement in perceived erectile function, and he has intensified physical activity, exercising nearly each day for about 45 min. He did not report any side effects from the change of the antihypertensive therapy.

Physical Examination

- Body weight decreased 1.5 kg from the first visit.
- No changes regarding others apparati.

Blood Pressure Profile

- Home BP (average): 128/80 mmHg
- Sitting BP: 130/80 mmHg
- Standing BP: 130/80 mmHg

Haematological Profile

- Fasting lipids: total cholesterol (TOT-C), 159 mg/dl; non-high-density lipoprotein cholesterol (non-HDL-C), 117 mg/dl; high-density lipoprotein cholesterol (HDL-C), 42 mg/dl; triglycerides (TG), 542 mg/dl
- Liver function tests: GOT, 33 U/L; GPT, 39 U/L; gamma-GT, 51 mg/dL (suggestive of a nonalcoholic fatty liver disease)

- CPK = 127 U/L

Current Treatment

- Therapeutic lifestyle
- Nebivolol 5 mg 1 tablet h. 8.00
- Telmisartan 40 mg 1 tablet h. 20.00

Treatment Evaluation

- Micronized fenofibrate 145 mg 1 cp h. 22.00

Prescriptions

- Maintenance of therapeutic lifestyle measures
- ABPM
- Liver ultrasonography
- Full haematochemistry

4.4 Follow-Up (Visit 3) at 1 Year

The patient reports a good adherence to the prescribed therapy and to the therapeutic lifestyle changes. He lost yet a bit weight. The glucose, lipid, and liver parameters strongly improved until normalization while reaching an optimal ABPM report without subjective side effects. The perceived impairment in erectile dysfunction is nearly disappeared.

Physical Examination

- Weight: 79.2 kg
- Height: 1.75 cm

- Body mass index (BMI): 25.8 kg/m^2
- Waist circumference: 93 cm
- Abdomen: normal, inferior margin of liver no more palpable below the costal margin

Haematological Profile

- Fasting plasma glucose: 92 mg/dL
- Fasting lipids: total cholesterol (TOT-C), 143 mg/dl; low-density lipoprotein cholesterol (LDL-C), 64 mg/dl; high-density lipoprotein cholesterol (HDL-C), 46 mg/dl; triglycerides (TG), 164 mg/dl
- Liver function tests: GOT 21 U/L, GPT 23 U/L, gamma-GT 32 mg/dL
- Serum uric acid: 5.1 mg/dL
- Renal function: urea, 12 mg/dl; creatinine, 1.0 mg/dL; creatinine clearance (Cockroft-Gault), 88.8 ml/min; estimated glomerular filtration rate (eGFR) (MDRD), 76 mL/min/1.73 m^2
- CPK = 152 U/L

Blood Pressure Profile

- Home BP (average): 130/76 mmHg
- Sitting BP: 128/84 mmHg (right arm); 130/84 mmHg (left arm)
- Standing BP: 130/80 mmHg at 1 min
- Twenty-four-hour BP: 125/82 mmHg; HR, 80 bpm
- Daytime BP: 128/85 mmHg; HR, 83 bpm
- Night-time BP: 118/72 mmHg; HR, 69 bpm

Twenty-four-hour ambulatory blood pressure profile is illustrated in Fig. 4.5.

Diagnostic Tests for Organ Damage or Associated Clinical Conditions

The liver ultrasound with ultrasound elastography image shows improvement of liver steatosis to a grade 1 fatty liver. IIEF-5 score = 18, suggesting a mild residual erectile dysfunction.

Current Treatment

- Therapeutic lifestyle
- Nebivolol 5 mg 1 tablet h. 8.00
- Telmisartan 40 mg 1 tablet h. 20.00
- Micronized fenofibrate 145 mg 1 cp h. 22.00

Treatment Evaluation Current Treatment

- Therapeutic lifestyle (confirmed)
- Nebivolol 5 mg 1 tablet h. 8.00 (confirmed)
- Telmisartan 80 mg 1 tablet h. 22.00 (if well tolerated)
- Micronized fenofibrate 145 mg 1 cp h. 22.00 (confirmed)

Prescriptions

- Periodical BP evaluation at home according to recommendations from current guidelines
- Standard 12-ECG and full haematochemistry once a year

Which will be the most useful diagnostic test to repeat during the follow-up in this patient?

Possible answers are:

1. Electrocardiogram
2. Echocardiogram

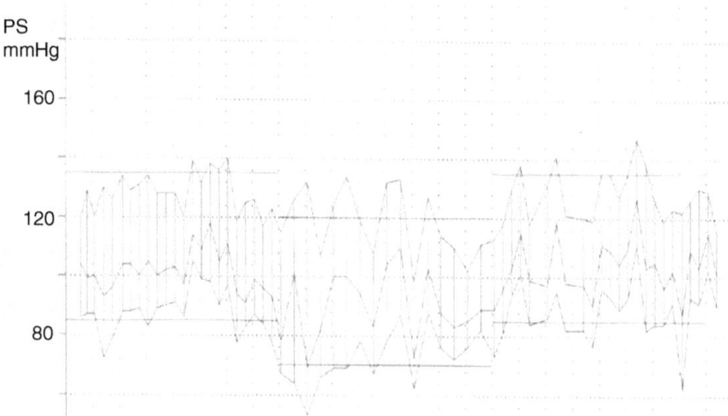

FIGURE 4.5 Patient post-treatment 24-h ambulatory blood pressure chart

3. Vascular Doppler ultrasound
4. Evaluation of renal parameters (e.g. creatininaemia, eGFR, ClCr, UACR)
5. Twenty-four-hour ambulatory BP monitoring

4.5 Discussion

Mendelian randomization data strongly suggests that hypertriglyceridaemia (HTG) causes atherosclerotic cardiovascular diseases and, after LDL cholesterol, is a secondary target to be considered. Fibrates (and in particular fenofibrate, because of its most favourable pharmacokinetic profile) are the best-established agents for TG level lowering and are generally used as first-line treatment of TG levels greater than 500 mg/dL [3]. Of course, before to begin a pharmacological treatment for hypertriglyceridaemia, it is useful to exclude all the secondary causes, like a wrong lifestyle and the negative effect of some drugs on lipid profile. It is well known that some antihypertensive drugs (and, namely, full dosed beta-blockers and thiazides) could impair plasma lipids, and, for this reason, these drugs have to be considered as second-line ones when treating a hypertriglyceridaemic patient [1]. Therefore, in the case of our patient, where the diet was already correct, the substitution of atenolol with a nonmetabolically interacting beta-blocker (like nebivolol) [4] and of the thiazide with telmisartan (an angiotensin receptor agonist with activating effect the peroxisome proliferator-activated receptor gamma (PPAR-g) [5]) improved triglyceridaemia without normalizing it (Fig. 4.6). The choice of telmisartan was also dictated by the possibility that it could have a parallel positive effect on NAFLD [6], an emerging cardiovascular risk factor, highly prevalent in hypertriglyceridaemic patients [3].

On the other side, the same drug changes significantly improved the perceived erectile dysfunction of the patient, often associated with the previously assumed drugs [7].

Of course, the management of the patient was not totally based on guidelines. For instance, the guidelines would have suggested to try to remove the beta-blocker and the thiazide, replacing them with a calcium antagonist. However, the patient already tried to remove the beta-blocker with reappraisal of a previously diagnosed tachycardia, while the choice of the sartan was based on the possibility that it could have some positive effects on his lipid metabolism.

Take-Home Messages

- Hypertriglyceridaemia is an emerging cardiovascular risk factor as well as nonalcoholic fatty liver disease (often associated with hypertriglyceridaemia)
- Some antihypertensive drugs, such as full-dosed old-generation beta-blockers and thiazides, are associated with an impairment of triglycerides.
- The same drugs are also often associated to impairment of erectile function in men.
- When treating hypertriglyceridaemic patients, it is relevant to choose antihypertensive drugs without metabolic interference with lipid metabolism

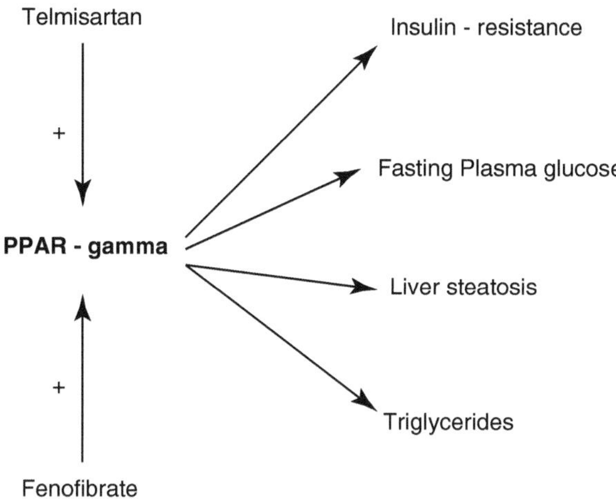

FIGURE 4.6 Effect of telmisartan and fenofibrate on some metabolic parameters

- Blockers of the renin-angiotensin-aldosterone system and calcium antagonists are usually preferred for the management of hypertensive patients with hypertriglyceridaemia. If a beta-blocker is needed, the more recent ones with less metabolic impact are preferred.

References

1. Mancia G, Fagard R, Narkiewicz K, Redon J, Zanchetti A, Bohm M, et al. 2013 ESH/ESC Guidelines for the management of arterial hypertension: the Task Force for the management of arterial hypertension of the European Society of Hypertension (ESH) and of the European Society of Cardiology (ESC). J Hypertens. 2013;31(7):1281–357.
2. Rosen RC, Riley A, Wagner G, Osterloh IH, Kirkpatrick J, Mishra A. The international index of erectile function (IIEF): a multidimensional scale for assessment of erectile dysfunction. Urology. 1997;49(6):822–30.

3. Brinton EA. Management of hypertriglyceridemia for prevention of atherosclerotic cardiovascular disease. Endocrinol Metab Clin North Am. 2016;45(1):185–204. doi:10.1016/j.ecl.2015.09.012.
4. Fergus IV, Connell KL, Ferdinand KC. A comparison of vasodilating and non-vasodilating beta-blockers and their effects on cardiometabolic risk. Curr Cardiol Rep. 2015;17(6):38. doi:10.1007/s11886-015-0592-x.
5. Cicero AF, Veronesi M, Prandin MG, Di Gregori V, Ambrosioni E, Borghi C. Effects of AT1 receptor and beta1 receptor blocking on blood pressure, peripheral hemodynamic and lipid profile in statin-treated hypertensive hypercholesterolemic patients. Fundam Clin Pharmacol. 2009;23(5):583–8. doi:10.1111/j.1472-8206.2009.00719.x.
6. Musso G, Gambino R, Cassader M, Pagano G. A meta-analysis of randomized trials for the treatment of nonalcoholic fatty liver disease. Hepatology. 2010;52(1):79–104. doi:10.1002/hep.23623.
7. Shah NP, Cainzos-Achirica M, Feldman DI, Blumenthal RS, Nasir K, Miner MM, Billups KL, Blaha MJ. Cardiovascular disease prevention in men with vascular erectile dysfunction: the view of the preventive cardiologist. Am J Med. 2016;129(3):251–9. doi:10.1016/j.amjmed.2015.08.038.

Chapter 5
Clinical Case 5: Patient with Essential Hypertension and Moderate Obesity

5.1 Clinical Case Presentation

Woman, 51 years old, never a smoker, overweight from childhood, and obese after the first (and unique) pregnancy. She is currently in menopause from a couple of months, with a tedious menopausal syndrome including flushing, excessive sweat, and hypertension. She has been treated with amlodipine 5 mg in the morning, but she stopped it because of the perception of flushing worsening.

Family History

Both parents of the patient were overweight, as well as her sister, 5 years younger. She has also a brother who is frankly obese. All the family is sedentary and has the tendency to eat much more energy than justified by their daily activity. However, no one in the family suffered from acute cardiovascular events. Her mother had a single gout attack. Her father is hypertensive and is complicated by left ventricular hypertrophy.

A.F.G. Cicero, *Hypertension and Metabolic Cardiovascular Risk Factors*, Practical Case Studies in Hypertension Management, DOI 10.1007/978-3-319-39504-3_5,

Clinical History

The patient has a relatively long list of cardiovascular risk factors: high blood pressure, atherogenic dyslipidaemia, impaired fasting glucose, ECG signs of left ventricular hypertrophy, and mild microalbuminuria, but no history of cardio- and cerebrovascular events. Overweight and a sedentary lifestyle also contribute to the cardiovascular risk profile of the patient, even if they are not included among the risk factors evaluated in the risk stratification of the ESH/ESC guidelines.

Physical Examination

- Weight: 85.9 kg.
- Height: 1.68 cm.
- Body mass index (BMI): 30.5 kg/m^2.
- Waist circumference: 101 cm.
- Respiration: auscultation of the chest reveals attenuated sounds, without murmurs and rubs.
- Heart sounds: regular rhythm, attenuated heart sounds, and no accessory murmurs.
- Resting pulse: regular, 58 bpm.
- Carotid arteries: no bruit on auscultation.
- Femoral and foot arteries: all pulses present and normosphygmic, even if not easy to be detected because of the body shape of the patient.
- Abdomen: largely globular, without other pathological signs.

Haematological Profile

- Haemoglobin: 13.9 g/dL
- Haematocrit: 42.6 %
- Fasting plasma glucose: 99 mg/dL

- Fasting lipids: total cholesterol (TOT-C), 174 mg/dl; low-density lipoprotein cholesterol (LDL-C), 97 mg/dl; high-density lipoprotein cholesterol (HDL-C), 47 mg/dl; triglycerides (TG), 148 mg/dl
- Electrolytes: sodium, 140 mEq/L; potassium, 3.9 mEq/L
- Serum uric acid: 5.7 mg/dL
- Renal function: urea, 21 mg/dl; creatinine, 0.9 mg/dL; creatinine clearance (Cockroft-Gault), 100.4 ml/min; estimated glomerular filtration rate (eGFR) (MDRD), 70 mL/min/1.73 m2
- Urine analysis (dipstick): gravity 1025, pH 6.6, no glucose nor sediments
- Albuminuria: 13 mg/24 h
- Liver function tests: GOT 28 U/L, GPT 31 U/L, gamma-GT 34 mg/dL
- Thyroid function tests: in the normal range

Blood Pressure Profile

- Home BP (average): 150/78 mmHg
- Sitting BP: 158/79 mmHg (right arm); 160/78 mmHg (left arm)
- Standing BP: 156/78 mmHg at 1 min
- Twenty-four-hour BP: 142/90 mmHg; HR, 68 bpm
- Daytime BP: 148/92 mmHg; HR, 74 bpm
- Night-time BP: 132/84 mmHg; HR, 65 bpm

Twenty-four-hour ambulatory blood pressure profile is illustrated in Fig. 5.1.

Twelve-Lead Electrocardiogram

The standard 12-lead ECG shows sinus rhythm (heart rate = 107 bpm) and small QRS complexes (3–4 mm in the limb leads, 6–7 mm in the precordial ones) (Fig. 5.2). Both before and after ECG execution, the heart rate measured at

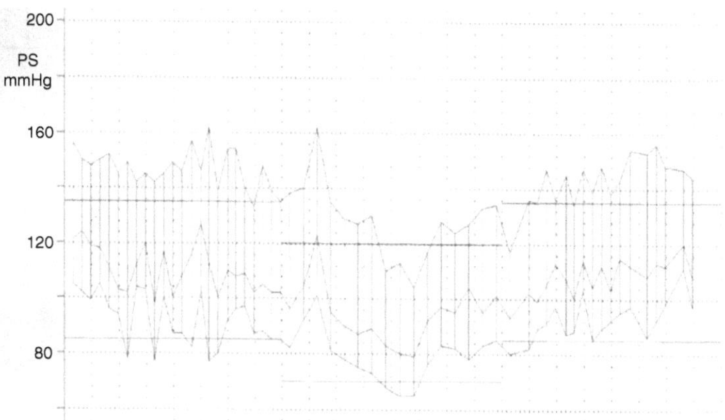

FIGURE 5.1 Baseline patient 24-h ambulatory blood pressure chart

the pulse was 50–60 bpm. The acceleration was probably due to the worrying of the patient seeing the nurse executing with difficulty the ECG because of her large breast.

Current Treatment

- None.

Diagnosis

Grade I hypertension in stage I obesity. Because of the presence of hypertension, large waist circumference, and mildly decreased HDL-C levels, the patient's clinical condition could also be considered as a metabolic syndrome, following the latest internationally harmonic diagnostic criteria (3 criteria on 5!) [1].

In the light of the available information, what is the estimated cardiovascular risk of the patient?

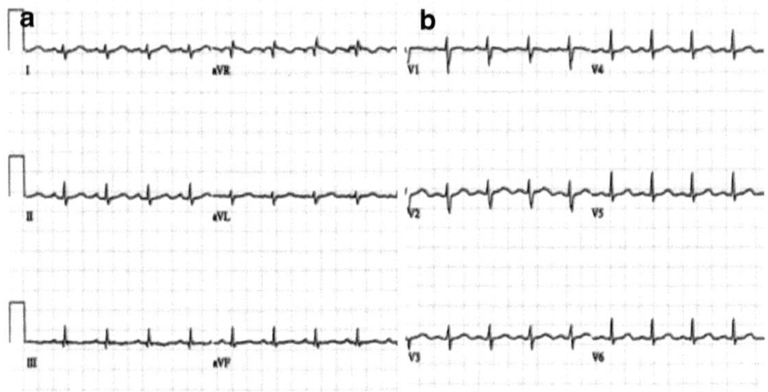

FIGURE 5.2 Patient baseline standard 12-lead ECG

Possible answers are:

1. Low
2. Medium
3. High
4. Very high

Global Cardiovascular Risk Stratification

The patient has one additional risk factor other than high blood pressure, so that she can be classified as a subject with moderate cardiovascular risk [2].

Treatment Evaluation

- Therapeutic lifestyle
- Phytoestrogens (soy extract 150 mg, containing genistein 30 mg and daidzein 30 mg)

Prescriptions

- Therapeutic lifestyle prescription, in particular the patient was instructed to follow the general indications of a moderately low carbohydrate Mediterranean diet, increasing the intake of vegetables and reducing as possible the consumption of salt. Moreover, she was also encouraged to increase her physical activity by walking briskly for 20–30 min, three to five times per week, or by cycling.
- Standard Echocardiography

5.2 Follow-Up (Visit 1) at 6 Weeks

The patient is satisfied because of the effect of phytoestrogens on flushing and sweating, but she said that the prescribed diet was not too different from the one she followed before, and she had not been able to increase her physical activity because of no habit to walk briskly.

Physical Examination

- Overall unchanged, when compared with the previous visit

Blood Pressure Profile

- Home BP (average): 148/78 mmHg
- Sitting BP: 154/78 mmHg
- Standing BP: 153/78 mmHg

Current Treatment

- Therapeutic lifestyle
- Phytoestrogens

Diagnostic Tests for Organ Damage or Associated Clinical Conditions

The standard echocardiography did not show any specific pathological signs. However, the quality of the exam was not good because of the patient's breasts and tachycardia during the test.

Diagnosis

Grade I hypertension in stage I obesity. Because of the presence of hypertension, large waist circumference, and mildly decreased HDL-C levels, the patient's clinical condition could also be considered as a metabolic syndrome, following the ATP III criteria (3 criteria on 5!) [1].

In the light of the available information, what is the estimated cardiovascular risk of the patient?

Possible answers are:

1. Low
2. Medium
3. High
4. Very high

Global Cardiovascular Risk Stratification

Since nothing has changed from a clinical point of view, the patient remains with one additional risk factors other than high blood pressure, which means that she can be classified as a subject with moderate cardiovascular risk [2].

Which is the best therapeutic option in this patient at this step?

Possible answers are:

1. Start with a dihydropyridinic calcium antagonist.
2. Start with a beta-blocker.
3. Start with a thiazide diuretic.
4. Start with an ACE inhibitor.
5. Start with an ARB.

Treatment Evaluation

- Therapeutic lifestyle
- Phytoestrogens
- Telmisartan 80 mg 1 tablet h 8.00

Prescriptions

- Intensification of therapeutic lifestyle measures: the patient has been prescribed a dietology visit and will be followed by a personal trainer to gradually increase the physical activity.

5.3 Follow-Up (Visit 2) at 3 Months

The patient reports improvement in home BP values without subjective side effects. She has began a low-carb high-protein diet since a couple of weeks with some weight loss, but she admits not to have followed the prescription about physical activity.

Physical Examination

- Body weight decreased 4.2 kg from the first visit.
- No changes as it regards other apparati.

Blood Pressure Profile

- Home BP (average): 136/76 mmHg
- Sitting BP: 142/80 mmHg
- Standing BP: 140/78 mmHg

Current Treatment

- Therapeutic lifestyle
- Phytoestrogens
- Telmisartan 80 mg 1 tablet h 8.00

Treatment Evaluation

- No drug has been modified.
- No drug dose has been changed.

Prescriptions

- Maintenance of therapeutic lifestyle measures
- Full haematochemistry and urinalysis

5.4 Follow-Up (Visit 3) at 1 Year

The patient reports a good adherence to the prescribed therapy and to a balanced Mediterranean diet (but she continues being sedentary). She has lost 18 kg after the low-carb high-protein diet and she recovered 2 kg during the normalization diet. The glucose, lipid, and liver parameters strongly improved until normalization with further improvement in home BP values without subjective side effects.

Physical Examination

- Weight: 69.4 kg
- Height: 1.68 cm
- Body mass index (BMI): 24.6 kg/m^2
- Waist circumference: 89 cm
- Abdomen: normal

Haematological Profile

- Fasting plasma glucose: 91 mg/dL
- Fasting lipids: total cholesterol (TOT-C), 161 mg/dl; low-density lipoprotein cholesterol (LDL-C), 91 mg/dl; high-density lipoprotein cholesterol (HDL-C), 52 mg/dl; triglycerides (TG), 88 mg/dl
- Liver function tests: GOT 19 U/L, GPT 17 U/L, gamma-GT 21 mg/dL
- Serum uric acid: 5.3 mg/dL
- Renal function: urea, 18 mg/dl; creatinine, 0.8 mg/dL; creatinine clearance (Cockroft-Gault), 90.6 ml/min; estimated glomerular filtration rate (eGFR) (MDRD), 80 mL/min/1.73 m2
- Urine analysis (dipstick): gravity 1025, pH 6.5, no glucose nor sediments
- Albuminuria: <10 mg/24 h

Blood Pressure Profile

- Home BP (average): 120/78 mmHg
- Sitting BP: 130/82 mmHg (right arm); 128/82 mmHg (left arm)
- Standing BP: 128/80 mmHg at 1 min
- Twenty-four-hour BP: 113/72 mmHg; HR, 66 bpm
- Daytime BP: 130/74 mmHg; HR, 71 bpm
- Night-time BP: 109/61 mmHg; HR, 53 bpm

Twenty-four-hour ambulatory blood pressure profile is illustrated in Fig. 5.3.

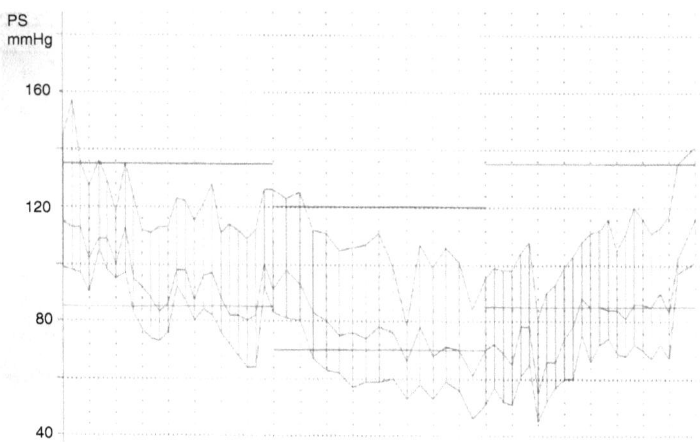

FIGURE 5.3 Patient post-treatment 24-h ambulatory blood pressure chart

Diagnostic Tests for Organ Damage or Associated Clinical Conditions

The patient was not further investigated for organ damage, since ECG, echocardiogram, and renal function were normal and blood pressure and body weight had been optimized.

Current Treatment

- Therapeutic lifestyle
- Telmisartan 1 tablet h. 8.00

Treatment Evaluation

- Therapeutic lifestyle (confirmed)
- Telmisartan 1 tablet h. 8.00 (confirmed), with dosage that could be halved during the summer if patient will suffer from orthostatic hypotension

Prescriptions

- Periodical BP evaluation at home according to recommendations from current guidelines
- Standard visit once a year, in particular, if body weight will increase again

5.5 Discussion

Obesity (space) is currently one of the greatest public health issues worldwide. However, even though its known deleterious effects on the cardiovascular system and its association with numerous cardiovascular diseases (CVD), recent findings leading to the development of concepts such as metabolically healthy obesity, the obesity paradox, and protective subcutaneous fat depots have raised a lively debate on the disparate effects of obesity on health outcomes [3].

The clinical case here described is an overall metabolically healthy obese patient, who developed hypertension after menopause. Therefore, menopause transformed a metabolically healthy obese patient in a mild metabolic syndrome patient.

Despite our efforts, the patient did not improve her physical activity, and a standard energy reduction did not induce a significant decrease in her body weight.

The phytoestrogen supplementation improved the patient's perceived quality of life, and it could exert some positive effects on the endothelial function of metabolic syndrome patients [4].

On the other side, a short-term low-carb high-protein diet could induce an impressive decrease in body weight and related anthropometric and metabolic parameters that remains even after 6 months [5], as seen in our patient.

As it regards the choice of the antihypertensive treatment, in this kind of patients, the guidelines suggest to prefer metabolically neutral drugs, like renin-angiotensin-aldosterone system blocking drug and/or calcium antagonists, maintaining thiazides or beta-blockers as second choices, when not strictly required [2].

In particular, telmisartan has been deeply investigated in obese patients, because its positive metabolic effects on lipid and glucose metabolism mediated by its activating effect on the peroxisome proliferator-activated receptor (space) gamma (PPAR-g) seems to be also associated to a redistribution of body fat from the visceral compartment to the subcutaneous one [6] (Fig. 5.4).

With the obtained body weight and blood pressure values, probably the prescribed antihypertensive drug could be stopped. However, the patient tolerated it very well and she does not experience any episode of hypotension, so no reason exists to interrupt it. However, the dosage could be reduced during the summer time in case of excessive weakness or hypotension.

Given the patient's family history and her lack of will to improve her physical activity, it is possible that she will recover (at least a part of) her original body weight, and,

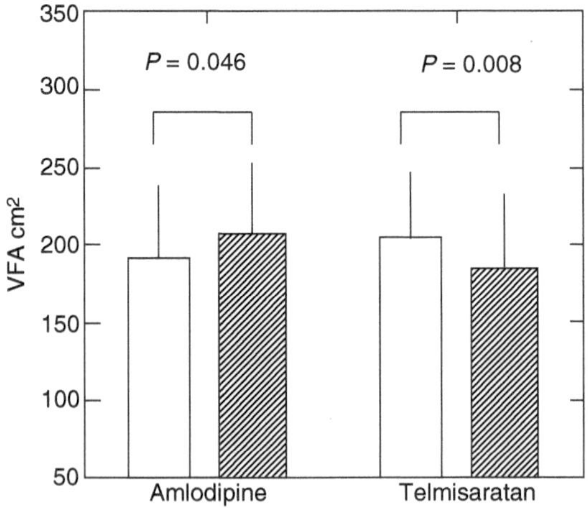

FIGURE 5.4 Comparison of the effect of telmisartan and amlodipine on visceral fat area in metabolic syndrome patients (Modified from [7])

consequently, the blood pressure could increase as well. This is the main reason for which the patient has to be scheduled for further control visits.

Take-Home Messages

- Obesity is usually associated with increased cardiovascular disease risk; however metabolically healthy subjects exist whose risk is inferior or similar to the one of nonobese subjects.
- Menopause could increase the risk associated with metabolically healthy obesity with the incidence of hypertension.
- If the intensification of dietary measures and physical activity are not possible or not able to improve body weight and blood pressure, thus an antihypertensive treatment is required.
- When treating obese patients, it is relevant to choose antihypertensive drugs without metabolic interference with glucose and lipid metabolism, nor body weight.
- Blockers of the renin-angiotensin-aldosterone system or calcium antagonists are usually preferred for the management of hypertensive patients with metabolic comorbidities.

References

1. Alberti KG, Eckel RH, Grundy SM, Zimmet PZ, Cleeman JI, Donato KA, Fruchart JC, James WP, Loria CM, Smith Jr SC. Harmonizing the metabolic syndrome: a joint interim statement of the International Diabetes Federation Task Force on Epidemiology and Prevention; National Heart, Lung, and Blood Institute; American Heart Association; World Heart Federation; International Atherosclerosis Society; and International Association for the Study of Obesity. Circulation. 2009;120:1640–5.
2. Mancia G, Fagard R, Narkiewicz K, Redon J, Zanchetti A, Bohm M, et al. 2013 ESH/ESC Guidelines for the management of

arterial hypertension: the Task Force for the management of arterial hypertension of the European Society of Hypertension (ESH) and of the European Society of Cardiology (ESC). J Hypertens. 2013;31(7):1281–357.
3. Kim SH, Després JP, Koh KK. Obesity and cardiovascular disease: friend or foe? Eur Heart J. 2015;pii:ehv509 [Epub ahead of print].
4. Irace C, Marini H, Bitto A, Altavilla D, Polito F, Adamo EB, Arcoraci V, Minutoli L, Di Benedetto A, Di Vieste G, de Gregorio C, Gnasso A, Corrao S, Licata G, Squadrito F. Genistein and endothelial function in postmenopausal women with metabolic syndrome. Eur J Clin Invest. 2013;43(10):1025–31.
5. Cicero AF, Benelli M, Brancaleoni M, Dainelli G, Merlini D, Negri R. Middle and long-term impact of a very low-carbohydrate ketogenic diet on cardiometabolic factors: a multi-center, cross-sectional, clinical study. High Blood Press Cardiovasc Prev. 2015;22(4):389–94.
6. Murakami K, Wada J, Ogawa D, Horiguchi CS, Miyoshi T, Sasaki M, Uchida HA, Nakamura Y, Makino H. The effects of telmisartan treatment on the abdominal fat depot in patients with metabolic syndrome and essential hypertension: Abdominal fat Depot Intervention Program of Okayama (ADIPO). Diab Vasc Dis Res. 2013;10(1):93–6.
7. Shimabukuro M, Tanaka H, Shimabukuro T. Effects of telmisartan on fat distribution in individuals with the metabolic syndrome. J Hypertens. 2007;25(4):841–8.

Chapter 6
Clinical Case 6: Adult Patient with Hypertension and Gout

6.1 Clinical Case Presentation

Man, 54 years old, ex-smoker since 20 years (25 smoked cigarettes for 15 years), mildly overweight, and hypertensive since 10 years. He began to be pharmacologically treated with antihypertensive drugs from the age of 50: his doctor prescribed him hydrochlorothiazide 25 mg per day. Initially, he tried atenolol 50 mg, but he had to stop it because of perceived decrease in sexual performances. Three months ago he suffered from a gout attack that resolved in a couple of weeks. Then, he was treated with allopurinol 300 mg ½ tablet per day which was not very well tolerated because of gastrointestinal discomfort. Recently, he came to our hypertension clinic for a general checkup because his blood pressure seems to be totally out of control.

Family History

The patient's father suffered from numerous episodes of gout and ~~he~~ died at the age of 69 because of an ischemic stroke. The mother is yet living, 91 y.o., not hypertensive nor diabetic. He has an older brother, 60 y.o., affected by chronic obstructive pulmonary disease, being yet a heavy smoker (30 cigarettes/day).

A.F.G. Cicero, *Hypertension and Metabolic Cardiovascular Risk Factors*, Practical Case Studies in Hypertension Management, DOI 10.1007/978-3-319-39504-3_6,

Clinical History

The patient is in primary prevention for cardiovascular disease, but his blood pressure is uncontrolled by the current antihypertensive therapy. Moreover, he hardly tolerates the current urate-lowering therapy, though he has just been suffered from a gout attack. Hyperuricaemia also contributes to the cardiovascular risk profile of the patient, even if it is not included among the risk factors considered in the risk stratification of the ESH/ESC guidelines. Furthermore, no one has ever prescribed him a therapeutic modification of the lifestyle aimed at reducing both blood pressure and serum uric acid, until now.

Physical Examination

- Weight: 86.9 kg.
- Height: 1.82 cm.
- Body mass index (BMI): 26.3 kg/m^2.
- Waist circumference: 105 cm.
- Respiration: auscultation of the chest reveals clear lung fields and no murmurs or rubs.
- Heart sounds: regular rhythm, no accessory rumours.
- Resting pulse: regular, 76 bpm.
- Carotid arteries: no bruit on auscultation.
- Femoral and foot arteries: all pulses present and normosphygmic.
- Abdomen: mildly globular, no other relevant signs.

Haematological Profile

- Haemoglobin: 14.3 g/dL
- Haematocrit: 44 %
- Fasting plasma glucose: 98 mg/dL
- Fasting lipids: total cholesterol (TOT-C), 176 mg/dl; low-density lipoprotein cholesterol (LDL-C), 92 mg/dl; high-

density lipoprotein cholesterol (HDL-C), 54 mg/dl; triglycerides (TG), 148 mg/dl
- Electrolytes: sodium, 140 mEq/L; potassium, 3.9 mEq/L
- Serum uric acid: 7.9 mg/dL
- Renal function: urea, 28 mg/dl; creatinine, 1.1 mg/dL; creatinine clearance (Cockroft-Gault), 94.5 ml/min; estimated glomerular filtration rate (eGFR) (MDRD), 76.0 mL/min/1.73 m^2
- Urine analysis (dipstick): gravity 1018, pH 6.7, no glucose nor sediments
- Albuminuria: 10 mg/24 h
- Liver function tests: GOT 20 U/L, GPT 22 U/L, gamma-GT 27 mg/dL
- Thyroid function tests: in the normal range

Blood Pressure Profile

- Home BP (average): 152/84 mmHg
- Sitting BP: 156/86 mmHg (right arm); 158/84 mmHg (left arm)
- Standing BP: 156/85 mmHg at 1 min
- Twenty-four-hour BP: 163/98 mmHg; HR, 79 bpm
- Daytime BP: 163/101 mmHg; HR, 82 bpm
- Night-time BP: 163/90 mmHg; HR, 70 bpm

Twenty four-hour ambulatory blood pressure profile is illustrated in Fig. 6.1.

The patient stated that he did not tolerate the ABPM, that his sleep was strongly disturbed by the measurements; and that he was often not able to stop his movements during the exam, since he is a bus driver.

Twelve-Lead Electrocardiogram

The standard 12-lead ECG show signs of left ventricular hypertrophy (Fig. 6.2). During the test, the patient declared to feel “a bit anxious”.

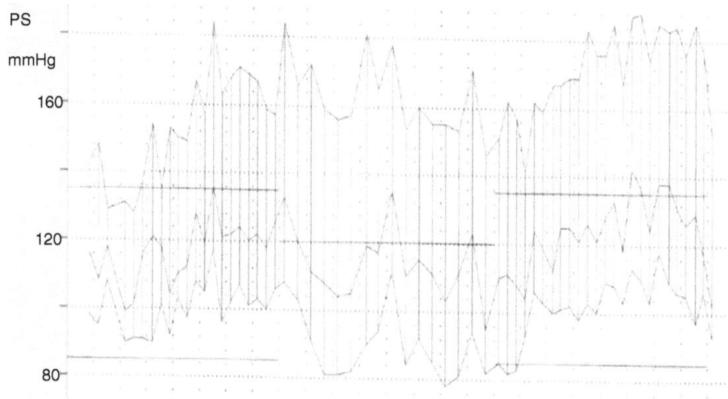

FIGURE 6.1 Baseline patient 24-h ambulatory blood pressure chart

Current Treatment

- Hydrochlorothiazide 25 mg 1 tablet h. 8.00
- Allopurinol 300 mg ½ tablet h. 8.00

Diagnosis

Grade I hypertension complicated by electrocardiographically diagnosed left ventricular hypertrophy, in hyperuricaemic patient with history of gout.

In the light of the available information, what is the estimated cardiovascular risk of the patient?

Possible answers are:

1. Low
2. Medium
3. High
4. Very high

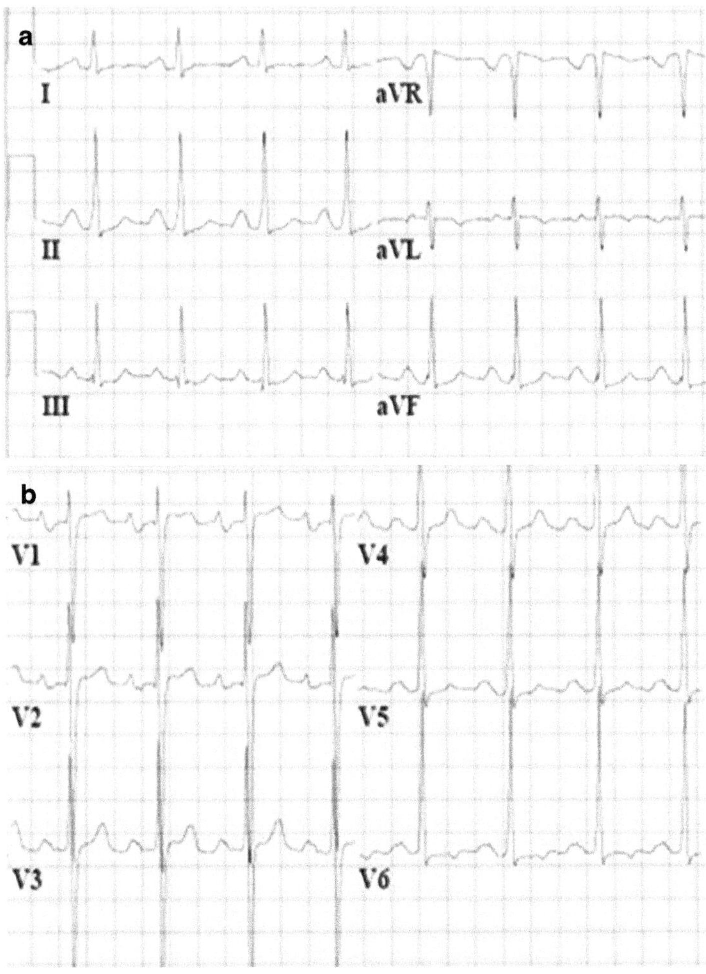

FIGURE 6.2 (**a**, **b**) Patient baseline standard 12-lead ECG

Global Cardiovascular Risk Stratification

The patient has more than left ventricular hypertrophy, an evident sign of target organ damage, so that he has to be classified as a subject with a high added cardiovascular risk [1]. Moreover, the subject has also high serum uric acid levels, not yet considered as a risk factor by the European guidelines, but independently associated with increased cardiovascular risk [2].

Which is the best therapeutic option for this patient at this step?

Possible answers are:

1. Add another drug class (e.g. dihydropyridinic calcium antagonist).
2. Add another drug class (e.g. beta-blocker).
3. Switch from the diuretic to a beta-blocker.
4. Switch from the diuretic to an ACE inhibitor.
5. Switch from the diuretic to an ARB.

Treatment Evaluation

- Losartan 100 mg 1 tablet h. 8.00 (instead of hydrochlorothiazide 25 mg) 1 tablet h. 8.00
- Allopurinol 100 mg tablet h. 8.00 (dosage mildly reduced)

Prescriptions

- Therapeutic lifestyle prescription, in particular the patient was instructed to follow the general indications of a Mediterranean low-energy diet, avoiding excessive intake of fat meats, organ meats, some seafood (anchovies, herring, sardines, mussels, scallops, trout, haddock, mackerel, and tuna), as well fructose and fructose-containing drinks (especially the ones rich in corn syrup).

6.2 Follow-Up (Visit 1) at 6 Weeks

The patient is pleased about the therapy, which he finds very well tolerable and acceptable. The gastrointestinal discomfort has been significantly decreased. Moreover, he claims that his

BP at home is "largely improved". He states to have put stronger attention to his diet, significantly reducing the content of salt and total energy, but to have continued eating seafood two times per week.

Physical Examination

- Overall unchanged, when compared with the previous visit. Body mass index and body weight are unchanged.

Blood Pressure Profile

- Home BP (average): 150/82 mmHg
- Sitting BP: 152/86 mmHg
- Standing BP: 152/84 mmHg

Current Treatment

- Therapeutic lifestyle
- Losartan 100 mg 1 tablet h. 8.00
- Allopurinol 100 mg tablet h. 8.00

Diagnostic Tests for Organ Damage or Associated Clinical Conditions

The carotid echo-colour Doppler ultrasound examination shows regular flow and normal intima-media thickness (Fig. 6.3).

Diagnosis

Grade I hypertension complicated by electrocardiographically diagnosed left ventricular hypertrophy, in hyperuricaemic patient with history of gout.

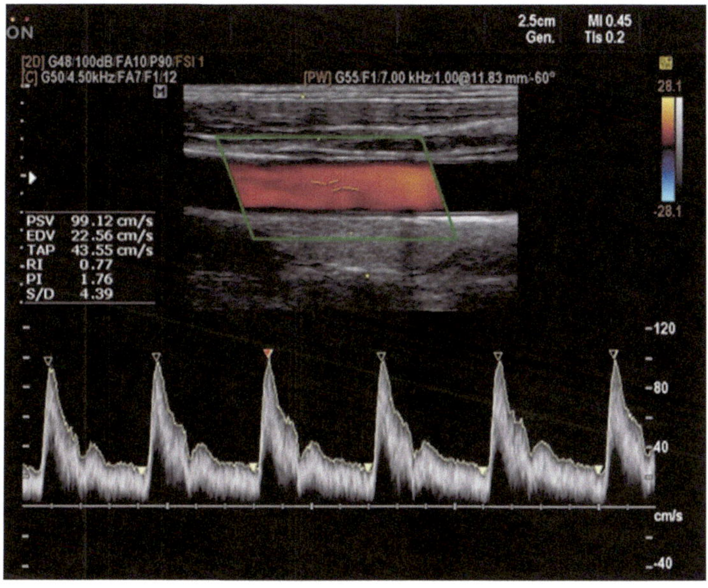

FIGURE 6.3 Patient carotid Doppler ultrasound

In the light of the available information, what is the estimated cardiovascular risk of the patient?

Possible answers are:

1. Low
2. Medium
3. High
4. Very high

Global Cardiovascular Risk Stratification

The patient continues being classified as a subject with a high added cardiovascular risk, because of uncontrolled BP and left ventricular hypertrophy, an evident sign of target organ damage [1]. Moreover, the subject has also high serum uric acid levels, not yet considered as a risk factor by the European guidelines, but independently associated with increased cardiovascular risk [2].

Which is the best therapeutic option for this patient at this step?

Possible answers are:

1. Add another drug class (e.g. dihydropyridinic calcium antagonist).
2. Add another drug class (e.g. beta-blocker).
3. Add another drug class (e.g. thiazide diuretic).
4. Add another drug class (e.g. alpha-blocker).
5. Switch from losartan to olmesartan.

Treatment Evaluation

- Therapeutic lifestyle
- Losartan 100 mg 1 tablet h. 8.00
- Amlodipine 5 mg 1 tablet h. 20.00 [added]
- Allopurinol 100 mg tablet h. 8.00

Prescriptions

- Intensification of the therapeutic lifestyle measures, with particular attention to physical activity
- Serum uric acid and renal function

6.3 Follow-Up (Visit 2) at 3 Months

The patient reports further improvement in home BP values without subjective side effects. He continues caring about diet and began to practise some physical activity.

Physical Examination

- Body weight decreased 2 kg from the first visit.
- No changes as it regards other apparati.

Blood Pressure Profile

- Home BP (average): 143/80 mmHg
- Sitting BP: 146/82 mmHg
- Standing BP: 146/80 mmHg

Haematological Profile

- Serum uric acid: 7.8 mg/dL
- Renal function: urea, 26 mg/dl; creatinine, 1.1 mg/dL; creatinine clearance (Cockroft-Gault), 74.9 ml/min; estimated glomerular filtration rate (eGFR) (MDRD), 70.0 mL/min/1.73 m^2 (85 kg)

Current Treatment

- Losartan 100 mg 1 tablet h. 8.00
- Amlodipine 5 mg 1 tablet h. 20.00
- Allopurinol 100 mg tablet h. 8.00

Which is the best therapeutic option for this patient at this step?

Possible answers are:

1. Increase the calcium antagonist dose.
2. Add another drug class (e.g. beta-blocker).
3. Add another drug class (e.g. thiazide diuretic).
4. Add another drug class (e.g. alpha-blocker).
5. Switch from losartan to olmesartan.

Treatment Evaluation

- Losartan 100 mg 1 tablet h. 8.00
- Amlodipine 10 mg 1 tablet h. 20.00 (dose increased)
- Febuxostat 120 mg tablet h. 8.00 (instead of allopurinol 100 mg)

Prescriptions

- Maintenance of the therapeutic lifestyle measures.
- Standard ECG.
- SUA level dosage.
- We would have prescribed a control 24-h ABPM, but the patient refused to repeat the exams. On the other side, the reliability of the first exam was low because of the low tolerability.

6.4 Follow-Up (Visit 3) at 1 Year

The patient reports a good adherence to the prescribed therapy and to the therapeutic lifestyle changes. He loses more weight. In particular, he tolerates much better febuxostat than allopurinol, with a strong improvement in serum uric acid.

Physical Examination

- Weight: 67.7 kg
- Height: 1.71 cm
- Body mass index (BMI): 23.3 kg/m^2
- Waist circumference: 92 cm
- Abdomen: normal, liver inferior border no more palpable below the costal margin

Haematological Profile

- Haemoglobin: 14.5 g/dL
- Haematocrit: 45 %
- Fasting plasma glucose: 91 mg/dL
- Fasting lipids: total cholesterol (TOT-C), 158 mg/dl; low-density lipoprotein cholesterol (LDL-C), 82 mg/dl; high-density lipoprotein cholesterol (HDL-C), 49 mg/dl; triglycerides (TG), 133 mg/dl
- Liver function tests: GOT 21 U/L, GPT 23 U/L, gamma-GT 26 mg/dL
- CPK = 158 U/L
- Electrolytes: sodium, 141 mEq/L; potassium, 3.8 mEq/L
- Serum uric acid: 5.3 mg/dL
- Renal function: urea, 23 mg/dl; creatinine, 1.0 mg/dL; creatinine clearance (Cockroft-Gault), 81.2 ml/min; estimated glomerular filtration rate (eGFR) (MDRD), 78.0 mL/min/1.73 m^2
- Urine analysis (dipstick): Gravity 1016, pH 6.8, no glucose nor sediments
- Albuminuria: 3 mg/24 h

Blood Pressure Profile

- Home BP (average): 134/78 mmHg
- Sitting BP: 136/82 mmHg (right arm); 135/80 mmHg (left arm)
- Standing BP: 134/80 mmHg at 1 min

Diagnostic Tests for Organ Damage or Associated Clinical Conditions

The patient standard ECG is reported in Fig. 6.4.

Although the voltage in all leads is normal as recorded, it is important to note the standardization seen at the end of the ECG tracing, which indicates that the limb leads were recorded at normal standard (1 mV = 10 mm or ten small boxes in height), while the precordial leads were recorded at half standard (1 mV = 5 mm or five small boxes in height). Hence the QRS amplitude as measured in the precordial leads needs to be doubled. Therefore, the R-wave amplitude in lead V5 is 24 mm, and the S-wave depth in leads V1 and V2 is 26 and 14 mm, respectively, for a total of 50 mm using S-wave depth in lead V1 + R-wave amplitude in lead V5 and 38 mm using S-wave depth in lead V2 + R-wave amplitude in lead in V5. This meets one of the criteria for left ventricular

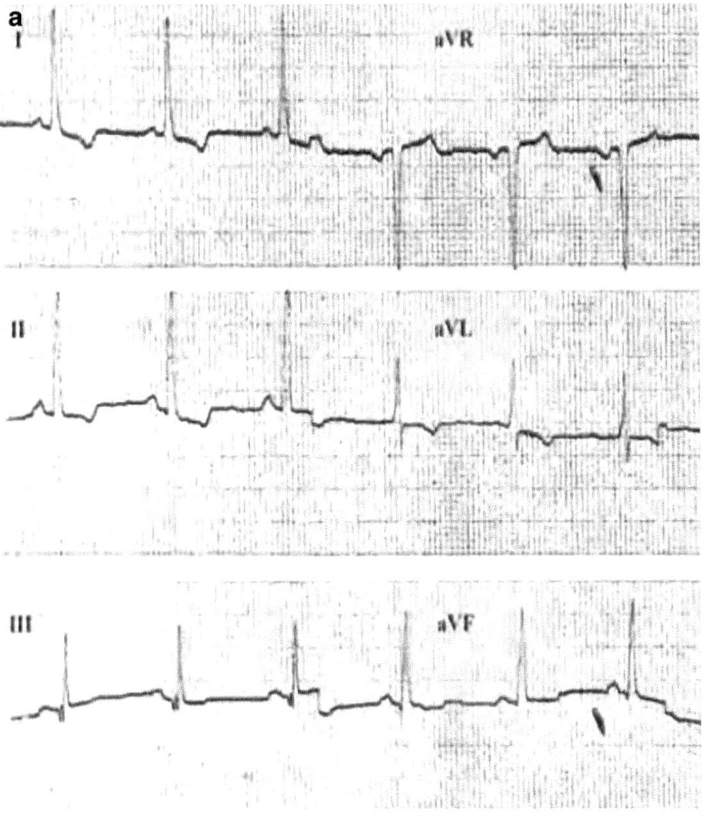

FIGURE 6.4 (**a**, **b**) Patient standard ECG

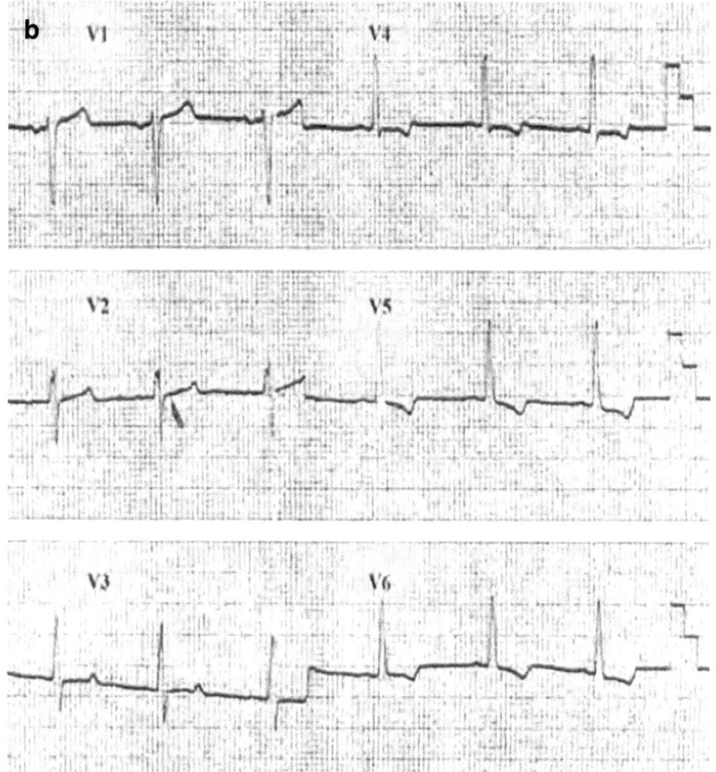

FIGURE 6.4 (Continued)

hypertrophy (S-wave depth in lead V1 or V2 + R-wave amplitude in lead V5 or V6 ≥ 35 mm). Typical ST-T wave changes associated with left ventricular hypertrophy seen in leads I, II, aVR (the positive T wave is actually inverted in this lead), and V4-V6 are present too.

Current Treatment

- Therapeutic lifestyle
- Losartan 100 mg 1 tablet h. 8.00

- Amlodipine 10 mg 1 tablet h. 20.00
- Febuxostat 120 mg tablet h. 8.00

Treatment Evaluation

- Therapeutic lifestyle (confirmed)
- Losartan 100 mg 1 tablet h. 8.00 (confirmed)
- Amlodipine 10 mg 1 tablet h. 20.00 (confirmed)
- Febuxostat 120 mg tablet h. 8.00 (confirmed)

Prescriptions

- Periodical BP evaluation at home according to recommendations from current guidelines.
- Standard 12-ECG once a year

6.5 Discussion

The relevance of elevated plasma levels of serum uric acid (SUA) in patients with cardiovascular disease was historically described two centuries century ago when Alexander Heig published a paper dealing with the causative role of hyperuricaemia in patients with hypertension and several other diseases [3]. More recently, a remarkable number of epidemiological and experimental studies have demonstrated that hyperuricaemia and gout are strongly related with hypertension, metabolic syndrome, chronic kidney disease, and cardiovascular disease [4]. On the other side, reducing the SUA level seems to be associated with a reduced cardiovascular risk [5]. The mechanism involved in these favourable effects could be the prevention of the oxidative stress linearly associated with the biochemical process which leads to uric acid formation [6].

The clinical case here described is common in general practice. High blood pressure and hyperuricaemia are strongly co-prevalent in general population, but high SUA levels could be predictors of hypertension and of left ventricular hypertrophy [7].

As it regards the choice of the antihypertensive treatment, in this kind of patients, the guidelines suggest to prefer metabolically neutral drugs, like renin-angiotensin-aldosterone system blocking drug and/or calcium antagonists, maintaining thiazides or beta-blockers as second choices, when not strictly required [2]. In particular, losartan seems to have a specific SUA lowering effect [8].

As it regards the choice of the SUA-reducing drug, given the low tolerability of allopurinol and the scarce efficacy of the low dose used, a more selective xanthine oxidase inhibitor, febuxostat, has been chosen, since it appeared to be better tolerated and more efficacious, as expected by the available data from clinical practice [9] (Fig. 6.5). The choice to directly use a high dose of febuxostat in this patient was related to the previous lack of efficacy of a low dose of allopurinol.

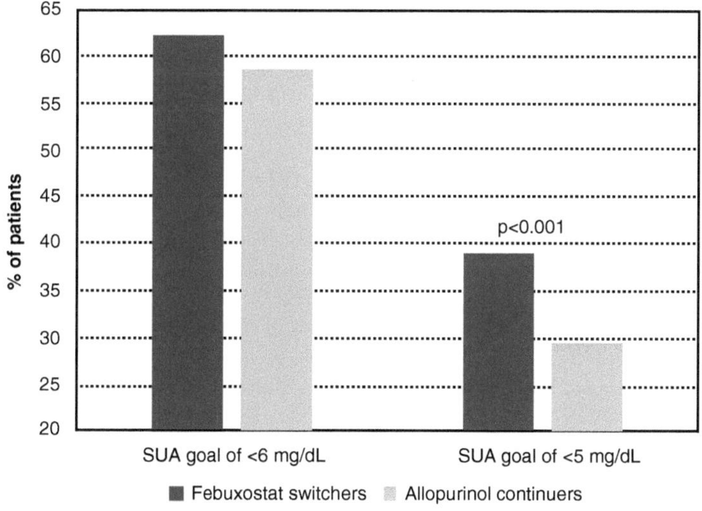

Figure 6.5 Improvement in SUA level switching from allopurinol to febuxostat in clinical practice (Modified from [9])

Take-Home Messages

- Hyperuricaemia is highly prevalent in general population, and it could increase the risk to develop hypertension and make its control more difficult.
- The overlapping of hyperuricaemia with hypertension strongly increases the risk to develop hypertension-related complication (in particular cardiovascular events).
- Therapeutic lifestyle can significantly improve both metabolic syndrome and blood pressure control.
- When treating hyperuricaemic patients, it is relevant to choose antihypertensive drugs without interference with uric acid metabolism.
- Among antihypertensive drugs, probably only losartan is associated with a mild improvement in serum uric acid, while full-dosed thiazides could impair it.

References

1. Mancia G, Fagard R, Narkiewicz K, Redon J, Zanchetti A, Bohm M, et al. 2013 ESH/ESC Guidelines for the management of arterial hypertension: the Task Force for the management of arterial hypertension of the European Society of Hypertension (ESH) and of the European Society of Cardiology (ESC). J Hypertens. 2013;31(7):1281–357.
2. Borghi C. The role of uric acid in the development of cardiovascular disease. Curr Med Res Opin. 2015;31 Suppl 2:1–2.
3. Galassi FM, Borghi C. A brief history of uric acid: from gout to cardiovascular risk factor. Eur J Intern Med. 2015;26:373.
4. Borghi C, Rosei EA, Bardin T, Dawson J, Dominiczak A, Kielstein JT, Manolis AJ, Perez-Ruiz F, Mancia G. Serum uric acid and the risk of cardiovascular and renal disease. J Hypertens. 2015;33:1729–41.
5. MacIsaac RL, Salatski J, Higgins P, Walters MR, Padmanabjan S, Dominiczak AF, Touyz RM, Dawson J. Allopurinol and cardiovascular outcomes in adults with hypertension. Hypertension. 2016;67:535–40.

6. Borghi C, Desideri G. Urate-lowering drugs and prevention of cardiovascular disease: the emerging role of xanthine oxidase inhibition. Hypertension. 2016;67(3):496–8.
7. Cicero AF, Rosticci M, Tocci G, Bacchelli S, Urso R, D'Addato S, Borghi C. Serum uric acid and other short-term predictors of electrocardiographic alterations in the Brisighella Heart Study cohort. Eur J Intern Med. 2015;26(4):255–8.
8. Smink PA, Bakker SJ, Laverman GD, Berl T, Cooper ME, de Zeeuw D, LambersHeerspink HJ. An initial reduction in serum uric acid during angiotensin receptor blocker treatment is associated with cardiovascular protection: a post-hoc analysis of the RENAAL and IDNT trials. J Hypertens. 2012;30(5):1022–8.
9. Altan A, Shiozawa A, Bancroft T, Singh JA. A Real-World Study of Switching From Allopurinol to Febuxostat in a Health Plan Database. J Clin Rheumatol. 2015;21(8):411–8.